The Spe

Penguin Library of Nursing

General Editor
Michael Bowman

The Cardiovascular System
The Digestive System
The Endocrine System
The Female Reproductive System
The Neuromuscular System
The Respiratory System
The Skeletal System
The Urological System
The Special Senses

The Penguin Library of Nursing Series was created by
Penguin Education and is published by Churchill Livingstone.

T. A. Casey
H. N. Waller

The Special Senses

Churchill Livingstone

CHURCHILL LIVINGSTONE
Medical Division of Longman Group Limited

Distributed in the United States of America by
Longman Inc., 19 West 44th Street, New York,
N.Y. 10036 and by associated companies,
branches and representatives throughout
the world.

© Longman Group Limited, 1976

ISBN 0 443 01495 7

Printed in Great Britain

Contents

Editorial foreword

Nursing has undergone considerable change during the past decade. There have been many developments in medical science and technology, and nursing education must keep pace with these changes, not merely in principle, but in terms of the nurse's attitude and approach. These changes primarily stem from the move towards caring for the patient in the context of his entire personality – the concept of total patient care. This concept was originally underlined in the 1962 Experimental Syllabus of Training and has subsequently been mirrored with greater emphasis in the 1969 Syllabus.

The education of the nurse, as voiced nationally and professionally in this decade, has merited prominence; this is certainly underlined in the recent *Report of the Committee on Nursing* (Briggs). It now appears likely that the once rather mythical education of the nurse is now approaching reality and fulfilment. For too long there has been conflict between the service needs of the hospital and the education of the nurse.

These require effective marriage if student satisfaction and general job satisfaction of the officers concerned and, perhaps most important of all, good patient care are all to be achieved. It is hoped that this series of textbooks will go some way towards helping students achieve a better understanding, in a more interesting way, of what this concept of total patient care is all about.

The series consists of nine books; together, these books make up an integrated whole, although each can be used in isolation. Each book embraces developmental embryology, applied anatomy and physiology, pathology, treatment, nursing care, social aspects and rehabilitation of the patient. In addition, each book contains a comprehensive list of further reading for the nurse.

It is hoped that students will find much pleasure in reading these books.

Michael Bowman,
Principal, Education Division, Hendon Group Training School,
Examiner to the General Nursing Council for England and Wales.

Introduction

In this book, the special senses of sight, hearing, taste and smell are all included. The infant makes his first contacts and becomes oriented in the world through these senses.

For many years, diseases connected with these senses were treated by the same specialist in the same hospital. As the importance of infection became appreciated, it was felt wiser to treat eye conditions, which were often uninfected, quite separately from diseases of the throat, nose or ears, which were often highly infectious. The two specialities are now usually separate, in different wards, often in different hospitals. Ophthalmology is closely associated with general medicine and neurosurgery, while ear, nose and throat surgeons work with general surgeons in the treatment of malignant disease and with plastic surgeons in the treatment of fractures of the face.

An absolute divorce has, however, not taken place between the two specialities. The pathology of one region can often be involved in the pathology of another. The eye, with its bony cavity, the orbit, is intimately related to the sinuses, and fractures of the orbit frequently trap eye muscles, so joint interference is necessary.

Eye surgeons and ear surgeons both make use of the operating microscope, and this has led to great advances in both fields.

Part one

The eye

Author's preface

For many years, eye nursing was ignored in the period of training and indeed the situation was little better with medical students. Ophthalmology, although a minority speciality, is no more difficult than others and the only explanation for its omission must be a lack of available time.

A basic understanding of eye nursing can be of immense value. Eye problems often arise in general wards, in industry and in casualty departments, and the nurse is often the first person to encounter them.

I know of a blind patient who came into a general ward for repair of his hernia. The doctors accepted his blindness but the nurse (who had recently attended eye lectures) asked a Registrar for an informal opinion. The patient subsequently had a corneal graft operation and was able to see again.

One of the most neglected conditions is that of early squint, and the nurse is often the first person the mother asks for advice.

In the preparation of the book I have had valuable help from the Visual Aids Departments of Hillingdon Hospital, Uxbridge, and the Queen Victoria Hospital, East Grinstead. My secretary, Miss Kathleen Streeter, has typed the manuscript on more than one occasion and Mrs Violet Hammond has given me valuable advice, while Anne Wade and Peter Tucker of Penguin Education have shown infinite patience and understanding.

T. A. Casey

Chapter 1   The anatomy and physiology of the eye

The eye is very similar to a camera in the way it works. When one looks at an object, an image of it is formed (upside down) on the *retina*, the very thin film at the back of the eye (Figure 1). This sends impulses to the brain, which turns the image the right way up. The eye has a diaphragm to cut down the amount of light entering it, and also a *lens* to bring a distant object into focus. The refraction of the light waves is carried out by the clear window at the front of the eye, the *cornea*.

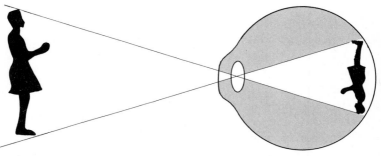

Figure 1 The principle of vision

The orbit

The eyeball (the *globe*) is suspended in the bony cavity known as the *orbit* by six strap-like muscles and various vessels and nerves. The relationships between the orbit and the surrounding structures are very important. Above the orbit is the *anterior cranial fossa* containing the anterior lobe of the brain. Below it is the *maxillary sinus*, laterally the *temporal fossa* and medially the *nasal fossa* and *ethmoid sinuses*. The medial wall is so thin that infection in the ethmoid sinuses can easily spread to the orbit, causing cellulitis. The floor of the orbit is also very thin, so that in a car accident, for example, it may fracture, and displace the globe downwards.

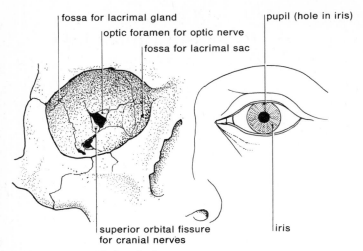

Figure 2 The orbit from in front

The orbit also contains the *lacrimal gland* which secretes tears, and the *lacrimal sac* which collects them. The latter is situated in the *lacrimal fossa* (Figure 2) and this is continuous with the *nasolacrimal duct* which enters the nose and ends under the *inferior turbinate* (see p. 68). There is also a good deal of orbital fat.

At the apex of the orbit is the optic canal which carries the *second cranial (optic) nerve* with its coverings of *dura, arachnoid* and *pia*. The *ophthalmic artery*, a branch of the internal carotid, is attached to the dura. On the lateral side of the optic canal is a comma-shaped fissure, the *superior orbital fissure*. This carries the third cranial (*oculomotor*) nerve, the fourth (*trochlear*) nerve, the sensory branches of the fifth (*trigeminal*) nerve, the sixth (*abducent*) nerve and sympathetic branches. Any brain tumours in this region, e.g. meningioma, can affect some or all of these important nerves.

The eye muscles

The six eye muscles originate from a tendinous ring which surrounds the optic foramen and part of the superior orbital fissure. The muscles fan out to become attached to the globe (Figure 3). These muscles control the movement of the globe, stimulated by the cranial nerves coming from the midbrain and the pons. The eyes move symmetrically, and the fields of

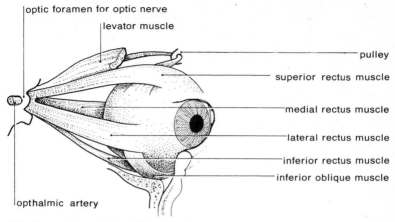

optic foramen for optic nerve
levator muscle
pulley
superior rectus muscle
medial rectus muscle
lateral rectus muscle
inferior rectus muscle
inferior oblique muscle
opthalmic artery

side view: outer wall of orbit removed

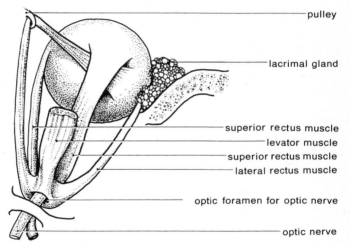

pulley
lacrimal gland
superior rectus muscle
levator muscle
superior rectus muscle
lateral rectus muscle
optic foramen for optic nerve
optic nerve

from above: roof of orbit removed

Figure 3 The eye muscles.
The levator muscle (cut in both diagrams) lifts the eyelid

vision overlap. The right eye obtains a slightly different view of an object from the left, giving man (alone among the animals) stereoscopic vision. If an eye muscle becomes defective, a *squint* results (one eye looks in or out or, more rarely, up or down).

The eye muscles

Name of muscle	Effect on eye
superior rectus	looks upwards
inferior rectus	looks downwards
medial rectus	looks towards the nose
lateral rectus	looks away from the nose
superior oblique	looks downwards and inwards and also causes rotation
inferior oblique	looks upwards and inwards and also causes anticlockwise rotation

The oblique muscles are unusual. The superior oblique is in two parts and runs through a pulley (the *trochlea*). Its nerve is the fourth (trochlear) nerve. The inferior oblique muscle is unusual in that it originates near the lacrimal sac, whereas the others arise from the apex of the orbit.

Nerve supply

The third cranial (oculomotor) nerve supplies all the eye muscles except the superior oblique, which is supplied by the trochlear nerve, and the lateral rectus, which is supplied by the sixth cranial (abducent) nerve. Thus, if the right eye is unable to turn inwards towards the nose, the medial rectus is paralysed, so this means that a branch of the third (oculomotor) nerve is involved.

The tissues of the eye

The eye is made up of three layers (Figure 4). The outermost layer is composed of fibrous tissue. The anterior part is the *cornea*, the transparent window at the front of the eye, and the posterior part is the *sclera*. This has the same composition as the cornea, but contains less water and is white and opaque. Under experimental conditions, the sclera can be made transparent by injecting it with water. The middle layer (often called the *uveal tract*) is in three parts, the *iris*, the *ciliary body* and the *choroid*. It is made up chiefly of blood vessels and pigment and is concerned with nutrition. The innermost layer is the *retina*, and is composed of nerve elements.

The cornea

This is transparent and has the shape of a meniscus lens, refracting the light rays. Water enters the cornea from tears and from the vessels in the sclera, but the cornea remains clear since its innermost lining, the

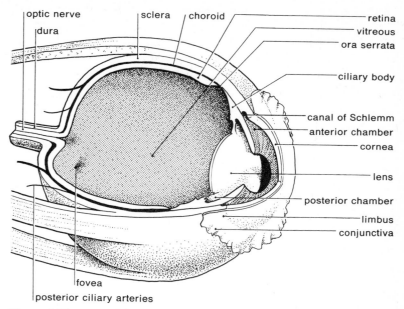

Figure 4 The parts of the eye

endothelium, acts as a pump and continuously takes water out of its substance. The cornea obtains oxygen from these sources as well as from the atmosphere and, if the oxygen is cut off, for example by the inaccurate fitting of contact lenses, clouding of the cornea occurs.

The sclera

This white, fibrous layer contains a posterior foramen for the optic nerve, and elsewhere is pierced by vessels and nerves. Its anterior part is covered by the *conjunctiva*. This is a membrane which extends over the sclera and lines the inner surfaces of the eyelids, but does not cover the cornea. When it is infected, the eye becomes red and sticky with a gritty feeling. However, this is not the only cause of red eye (see p. 26).

The iris

This is a thin circular disc with a hole in the centre which is known as the *pupil*. It consists of muscle, blood vessels and pigment, the last being concerned with the colour of the eyes. They may be blue, grey or brown and can vary in the same person with age.

The iris works like the diaphragm in a camera. It regulates the amount of light coming into the eye, with the pupil contracting in bright sunshine and dilating in the dark. Its musculature is controlled by the sympathetic nerves and by a branch of the third cranial nerve (the parasympathetic).

Drugs which dilate the pupil are known as *mydriatics*. Examples are *atropine*, *adrenaline* and *mydrilate*. Those which constrict the pupil are known as *miotics*, and examples are *pilocarpine* and *eserine*.

The ciliary body

This is continuous with the iris in front and with the choroid behind. As well as being made up of muscles, blood vessels and pigment, it also contains a lining of ciliary epithelium (which resembles a gland) and secretes the important fluid known as *aqueous humour*. This fills the space between the cornea and the iris and provides nutrition for them. It is very similar to the cerebrospinal fluid, draining into a venous sinus called the

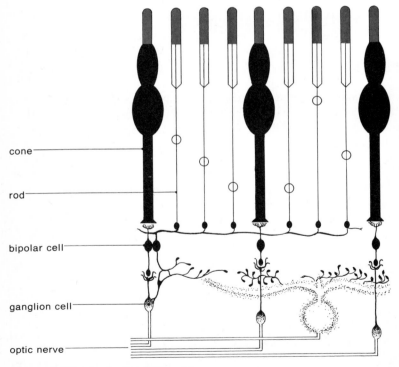

Figure 5 The visual cells of the retina

canal of Schlemm, which lies deep in the substance of the sclera at its junction with the cornea. This aqueous humour has been the subject of intense study recently, since *glaucoma* (see p. 32) is caused by disorders of its drainage. Glaucoma is responsible for 13 per cent of all blindness.

The choroid

This is the continuation backwards of the ciliary body and lies between the sclera and the retina. It is composed almost entirely of blood vessels which nourish the outer layer of the retina.

The retina

This is a delicately thin membrane composed of complicated nervous receptors (various types of nuclei and fibres) and blood vessels. In the living it is of a purplish-red colour but, if the eye is opened after death, the retina is found to be white. This is because the retina contains visual purple, which is bleached by light.

The visual cells of the retina are called *rods* and *cones* (Figure 5). They

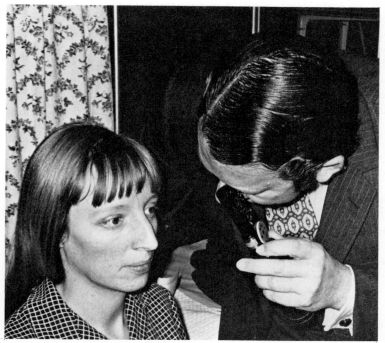

Figure 6 An ophthalmoscope

contain visual pigments which absorb certain wavelengths of light. In this process energy is released, causing an electrical impulse which results in the awareness of colour. The rods are chiefly concerned with night vision. If they are defective, there is difficulty in adjusting to the dark. There are three specific cone receptors for the colours red, blue and green. A colour such as yellow is perceived by stimulation of a mixture of cones.

Complete *colour blindness* is extremely rare (1 in 100 000 000 people). More common (especially in men) is *defective colour discrimination*, in which blue and yellow can be distinguished, but not colours in the blue–green area between them. Some eye diseases, such as cataract, can cause difficulty in judging colour. An example of this is the painter Turner, who avoided using colours at the blue end of the spectrum.

The vessels in the retina can be studied with an instrument known as an *ophthalmoscope* (Figure 6). Diseases such as hypertension and diabetes frequently cause abnormalities of the retina (see Chapter 3).

Tears

Men and elephants are said to be the only animals that cry. Tears are essential to preserve the transparency of the cornea. They are formed in the *lacrimal glands* in the upper and outer parts of the orbit (Figure 7) and, in equal amounts, by the mucus glands of the conjunctiva. Excess tears escape through channels in the eyelid margins and eventually enter the nose. They have a salty taste. Occasionally, in rheumatoid arthritis, tears may be defective, and they must be replaced by tear substitutes of saline, or methyl cellulose which does not evaporate easily.

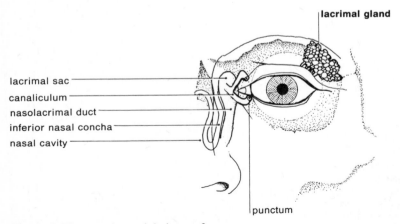

Figure 7 The secretion and drainage of tears

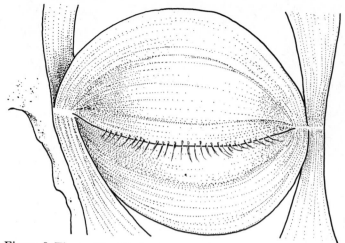

Figure 8 The eyelids with the skin removed showing the orbicularis muscle

The tears are pumped into the channels in the eyelid margins (the *canaliculi*) and then into the lacrimal sac and the nose by the massaging action of the eyelids. The eyelids are made up of two muscles. The *orbicularis oculi* is a circular muscle (Figure 8) which spreads on to the forehead and cheek, and is the muscle which contracts when the eyelids are tightly closed. It is supplied by the seventh cranial (*facial*) nerve. In facial palsy, this nerve is affected and such patients may sleep with their eyelids open. The other muscle is the *levator* muscle, which opens the eyelid. The eyelids have the dual function of protecting the eye both from excessive light and from irritating foreign particles. They may be thought of as windscreen wipers which keep the cornea clean and help to distribute tears across it.

Ophthalmology

For many years, diseases of any of the special senses were dealt with by the same specialist. But, about twenty-five years ago, following the development of antibiotics, *ophthalmology* became a separate speciality, associated with general medicine and neurosurgery. Ear, nose and throat specialists then tended to work more closely with general surgeons in the treatment of malignant disease and with plastic surgeons in the treatment of fractures of the face. However, close cooperation between the two divisions of the special senses is still necessary, as the orbit of the eye is

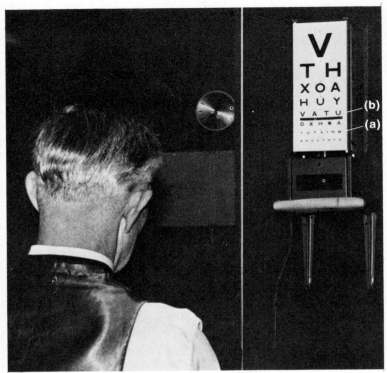

Figure 9 Testing visual acuity by Snellen's charts.
Ability to read line (*a*) at 6 metres represents normal vision (acuity = 6/6),
whilst ability to read line (*b*) at this distance is equivalent to being able to read
a car number plate at 25 yards

closely related to the sinuses, and tumours and abscesses from the latter
occasionally invade the orbit. Also, tears drain from the lacrimal sac into
the nose and the two divisions need to work together to check for a nasal
obstruction at the end of the nasolacrimal duct.

An ophthalmologist is also known as an *ophthalmic surgeon* or an *oculist*
(but not an optician, who is not medically trained and mainly tests for and
sells spectacles). The ophthalmologist, however, may also test for
spectacles and contact lenses. In out-patient clinics he treats eye infections
such as corneal ulcers and eye inflammations such as iritis. He supervises
the treatment of glaucoma and may assist a physician in the wards in

diagnosing disorders where there may be accompanying eye signs, such as in a brain tumour or in a difficult problem like sarcoid. In the operating theatre he will perform cataract and squint surgery, perhaps graft the cornea from a deceased donor to an eye that has been blinded, say from acid burns, and he may even use a laser to solder holes in detachment of the retina.

The role of the nurse in ophthalmology may be wide-ranging. A very important part of the work is to help allay the anxiety of patients and relatives by explaining procedures to them. For example, elderly cataract patients will be relieved to hear that they can get up the day after their operation and that only one eye is bandaged. Parents of children will also be relieved to hear that the eyes of their children will not be bandaged after squint surgery.

Other duties of the nurse may be to take *visual acuities* (of the smallest print the patient can read when seated six metres from a standard chart, Figure 9). The nurse may assist the ophthalmologist by removing corneal foreign bodies. She may also instil eye drops and ointment, and in some clinics nurses check eye pressures in patients with glaucoma and syringe the tear passages of patients with watering eyes.

Summary of nursing points

The nurse must appreciate the importance of the eye in the context of the personality as a whole. She should become thoroughly conversant with the development, structure and functions of the eye. She should also acquaint herself with the preparation of the patient for any special test or investigation that may be indicated. The nurse should also be clear on the emergency conditions of the eye, such as a foreign body in the eye, which require prompt first-aid measures.

A very important task of the nurse in ophthalmology is to allay her patients' anxiety and apprehension by explanation, support and reassurance.

Chapter 2   Disorders of the eye

In this chapter, a number of different but very important disorders of the eye are brought together. There are three main topics: the *red eye*, which is the most important eye affection, *cataract* and *glaucoma*, which together account for 45 per cent of the blindness in the Western world, and, finally, a section on *squint* and other diseases.

Red eye

This is very important, and demands urgent treatment. The nurse is often the first person to see the patient, whether in the casualty department, the works' dispensary, in the hospital wards or as a midwife. A knowledge of the differential diagnosis of red eye is thus of the utmost importance.

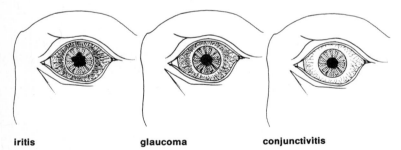

iritis   **glaucoma**   **conjunctivitis**

Figure 10 Causes of red eye

There are three main causes (Figure 10): *conjunctivitis* (inflammation of the outer eye), *acute iritis* (inflammation of the inner eye) and *acute glaucoma* (a congested, tense eyeball), in which there is an obstruction to the outflow of aqueous humour. A fourth, less usual cause is an *acute keratitis* (inflammation of the cornea). This presents as a *corneal ulcer*.

Acute conjunctivitis

The patient complains of a red eye and, on examination the inflammation, is found to have a characteristic distribution. It is generalized and is equally manifest in the *tarsal conjunctiva* (the conjunctiva lining the inner surface of the eyelids). This is in sharp contrast to iritis, where the redness is most marked at the corneal margin.

The blood and tissue cells fight the infection by producing an inflammatory discharge. This is usually most noticeable in the morning, when the eyelids are often glued together. The type of discharge depends on the severity of the infection; it may be *purulent*, *mucopurulent* or *catarrhal*.

The discomfort felt by the patient, often referred to as a 'gritty' feeling in the eye, is caused by the rubbing together of the tarsal conjunctiva and the conjunctiva covering the sclera.

There are a number of organisms which can cause the infection. In Britain, common ones are pneumococcus, staphylococcus, coliforms, streptococcus, *H. influenzae* and viruses. There are five main modes of infection:

1 Direct infection, either by intimate contact with an infected person or by using the same face towels, etc.;

2 Airborne infection by dust and droplets;

3 Waterborne infection through swimming pools;

4 From the unwashed hands of a surgeon, nurse or the patient himself;

5 Epidemics in hospital wards, industrial plants, homes for the aged (the mechanisms here are often obscure).

There is usually no pain in conjunctivitis, and this is an important point in differential diagnosis. Visual acuity is normal, and there is no photophobia (light sensitivity).

Catarrhal conjunctivitis

Most of us have been affected by this at some period of our lives. It occurs slightly more frequently in winter, and the common causal organisms are pneumococci and *H. aegyptius.*

A conjunctival swab must be taken, to identify the causative organism, and tests are then performed to determine the antibiotic to which it is sensitive. As this usually takes about 48 hours, drops of a broad-spectrum antibiotic are usually given immediately. A drug commonly used in ophthalmology is *chloramphenicol.* Resistance to it is unusual, since it is seldom used systemically, and allergic reactions are uncommon. It retains its activity for two weeks, which is long enough to treat most infections. Other less useful drugs are *neomycin* (which loses its activity after three days) and *penicillin* (which is very effective but frequently produces allergic reactions on the eyelids).

If chloramphenicol (or any other antibiotic) is given in the form of drops, these must be given frequently – every two hours, or every hour if the infection is severe. It is useless to give them only twice a day, as they are washed away by the tears. The method of administration is shown in Figure 11. In no circumstances must the dropper actually touch the eyelid. If more than one patient is affected in a ward or in a factory, each patient

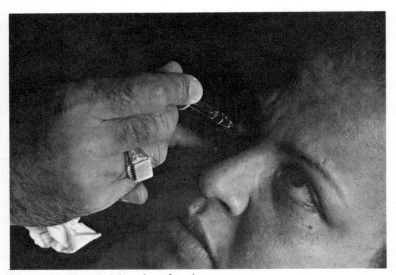

Figure 11 The administration of eyedrops

must have his own dropper. At night, chloramphenicol ointment is used, which keeps up the antibiotic concentration and also prevents the matting of the eyelids so commonly found in this condition.

The eye should never be covered, as the heat engendered by the patch forms an ideal culture medium for the organisms.

Ophthalmia neonatorum

This is now very rare. It is an inflammation of the eye in a newborn baby and, before the advent of antibiotics, was a common cause of blindness from secondary corneal ulceration. The baby picked up a purulent conjunctivitis from a gonococcal infection in the mother, during birth. On the rare occasions when this condition now occurs, the discharge should be wiped away, and antibiotic drops given at half-hourly intervals with systemic antibiotics.

The most common cause of eye infections in the newborn nowadays is a virus infection, *inclusion conjunctivitis*. Scrapings from the conjunctiva will enable a diagnosis to be made and the same virus will be isolated from the mother's cervix. Fortunately, this disease is not associated with corneal complications.

Trachoma

This is extremely rare in Britain, but in India and the Middle East it is responsible for millions of cases of blindness. The disease, associated with dust and insanitary living conditions, is a conjunctivitis caused by a virus, and it leads to secondary corneal scarring and *vascularization* (the ingrowth of vessels into the cornea). Although it is caused by a virus, it is just susceptible to antibiotics.

Acute iritis

The iris is the anterior part of the uveal tract, pierced by a central hole, the pupil. Inflammation may occur in different sites. If only the iris is involved, it is termed *iritis*; when the ciliary body is also affected, it is termed *iridocyclitis* and, if the choroid is involved, this is *choroiditis*. If all three are affected, the term *uveitis* is used.

The patient presents with a red eye, but the redness in iritis is quite typical. It is referred to as *ciliary* or *circumcorneal injection*. The maximum redness in iritis is at the margin of the cornea (see Figure 10), whereas in conjunctivitis the engorgement is spread evenly over the whole conjunctival surface.

The pupil is small and, if the iritis has been present for a few days, it may be irregular because of adhesions (*posterior synechiae*) to the underlying lens. In conjunctivitis, the pupil is normal. Vision is moderately affected because of the outpouring of white cells into the space between the cornea and the iris (the *anterior chamber*). In some cases this outpouring may be massive and pus develops in the anterior chamber. This is known as a *hypopyon* (Figure 12). The eyeball is tender and painful and this pain does not cease when the patient closes his eyes at night. Photophobia is common and is helped by dark glasses.

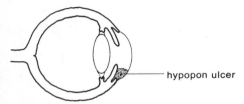

hypopon ulcer

Figure 12 Hypopyon ulcer

Unlike conjunctivitis, which eventually clears even without treatment, iritis lasts for months, and frequently damages vision. The complications include *secondary glaucoma* from the adhesions referred to above, and *secondary cataract* through impairment of lens nutrition.

Iritis is an inflammation, not an infection, i.e. microorganisms cannot be found on the iris. In our present inadequate state of knowledge it is considered to be an allergic or hypersensitivity reaction. It is frequently associated with certain systemic diseases – ankylosing spondylitis, sarcoid, Still's disease (in children), prostatitis and syphilis. In 70 per cent of cases, the aetiology of iritis is not determined; but when an association such as sarcoid is found, it must be treated vigorously with systemic steroids.

Treatment
Atropine and *corticosteroid* drops are the usual form of treatment, but they must not be used unless the diagnosis is certain. Atropine is disastrous if the red eye is actually due to acute glaucoma and, if cortisone drops are given for a corneal ulcer, the eye may perforate!

Atropine (1 per cent) paralyses the ciliary muscle and iris sphincter and allows relief from the pain due to spasm. It dilates the pupil and prevents adhesions between the iris and the lens. It is usually given three times daily. The nurse must be careful not to contaminate her fingers, since the dilated pupil cannot be counteracted and may last for two weeks.

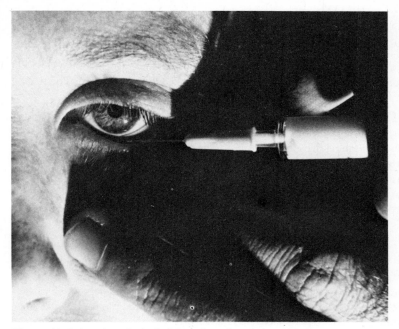

Figure 13 Subconjunctival administration of corticosteroid

Corticosteroids inhibit the inflammatory response and allow for spontaneous resolution. They must be administered as necessary to keep the eye white and quiet. *Maxidex* is a common proprietary preparation and is given every two hours. Ointment may be given at night to keep up the cortisone concentration during sleep. If the inflammation is very severe, the corticosteroid can be given subconjunctivally (Figure 13), and this may be supplemented by oral steroids, such as *prednisolone* (5 mg four times daily).

The eye may be made more comfortable and the photophobia relieved if the eye is kept closed by a pad. Hot spoon bathing was formerly used, but is of little value.

Sympathetic ophthalmia

This is a rare form of iritis which generally follows a perforating injury to one eye. Two to four weeks later, an inflammation starts in the other eye, and this is so persistent that both eyes may become blind. Treatment consists in removal of the injured eye and the use of corticosteroids to the 'sympathizing' eye.

Acute glaucoma

If a perforated appendix is the great emergency in general surgery, acute glaucoma is its counterpart in ophthalmology. *Glaucoma* is a rise in intraocular pressure just as hypertension is a rise in systemic blood pressure. There are two types, *acute* and *chronic* (or insidious). These are two quite distinct diseases and have completely different causes.

The patient with acute glaucoma (frequently a woman) presents with a red eye, whose redness is of the ciliary type, i.e. it is most marked at the corneo–scleral margin. In addition, the patient complains of pain around the eye and may be nauseated or even vomiting. Her vision is severely reduced, at times to 'perception of light' only. The symptoms may not always be quite so dramatic, in which case it is important to avoid any confusion with conjunctivitis. In iritis, the *intraocular pressure* (see p. 43) is sometimes raised.

The history of the patient will provide very valuable clues to diagnosis. The majority of patients who suffer an attack of acute glaucoma have warning signs such as periods of blurred vision, or seeing rings around street lights. This is because episodes of raised intraocular pressure cause mild oedema. This is more likely to happen when the pupil is dilated and drainage is restricted, such as at night, after a film or after an emotional shock.

The cause of acute glaucoma, unlike that of chronic glaucoma, is very simple to understand. The space between the cornea and iris (the *anterior chamber*) is too shallow and, when the pupil dilates, the drainage channels for aqueous humour are blocked off.

Treatment
It has already been stressed that incorrect treatment will be disastrous to vision. The aim of the treatment is primarily to constrict the pupil and so to disencumber the angle (Figure 14) of the anterior chamber. It entails

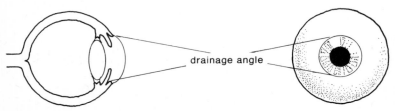

drainage angle

Figure 14 The drainage angle in acute glaucoma

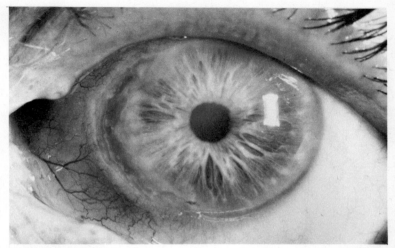

Figure 15 Corneal ulcer

giving *pilocarpine* (2 per cent every ten minutes for several hours), often combined with *eserine* (1 per cent). The formation of aqueous humour is prevented by giving *diamox* (*acetazolamide*) tablets (250 mg). Two tablets are given initially and later one tablet is given four times daily. Occasionally the diamox is given intravenously. If the intraocular pressure is not sufficiently reduced by this treatment, *glycerol* (1 ml per kg bodyweight) is given orally. Intravenous *mannitol* is given if the attack is severe. If these measures are unsuccessful in 24 hours, an operation will be needed to allow the aqueous humour to drain through the original channel under the conjunctiva. It should be noted that the other eye must also have miotic drops, since bilateral acute glaucoma may occur.

Acute keratitis

A corneal ulcer (Figure 15) is the most common manifestation of *acute keratitis* (inflammation of the cornea). Since the cornea is exposed throughout life to a succession of minor traumata, the normal conjunctival organisms may invade the cornea.

There are two main types of corneal ulcer:

1 The *marginal ulcer*. This is usually a bacterial ulcer, and it responds readily to local antibiotic drops.
2 The *dendritic ulcer*. This is a central ulcer usually caused by a virus.

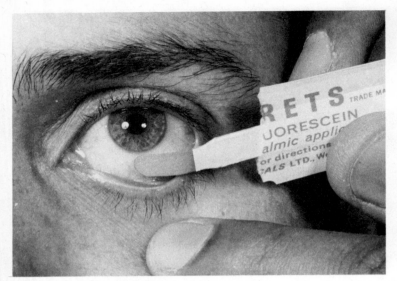

Figure 16 Staining with fluorescein

These infections are more frequent now than twenty years ago, although we do not know why. This ulcer is responsible for a good deal of unilateral blindness because it is often treated incorrectly. Unfortunately there is no satisfactory explanation for the mechanism by which the virus reaches the cornea. The *Herpes simplex* virus present in the skin around the eyes may give rise to a 'cold sore' when the patient is at a low ebb with influenza. Sometimes sunshine triggers an attack. Some cases of dendritic ulcer result from parents kissing their children's eyelids.

The patient presents with a red eye of the ciliary type. Mild pain is common as the epithelium of the cornea is denuded and the cornea has an extremely rich nerve supply. In mild cases, the visual acuity is only slightly affected. The diagnosis of early cases will be missed unless a vital stain such as fluorescein is instilled into the conjunctival sac. Alternatively this dye may be impregnated into sterile filter paper (Figure 16).

Treatment
An important point about the treatment of acute keratitis is that preparations of steroids and antibiotics should never be used since, although steroids help to reduce the inflammation for a few days, they also help the virus to multiply with the risk that the cornea may perforate. A

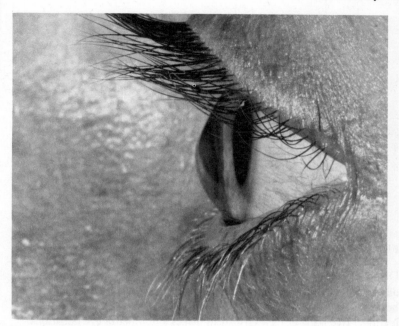

Figure 17 Keratoconus

new drug which is useful is *idoxuridine* (IDU), drops of which are given every hour until the epithelium ceases to stain with fluorescein. The process of *carbolization*, that is, painting the whole corneal surface with carbolic acid, has the effect of killing the epithelial cells (which quickly regenerate) and also of killing the virus. If the attack lasts for six to eight weeks, or if there are frequent recurrences, the cornea which carries the virus may be replaced by a cornea transplanted from a cadaver. This is a very successful form of treatment and is usually necessary for patients who have been injudiciously treated with steroids.

Corneal grafting

This operation was first performed successfully over a hundred years ago on a pet gazelle. Operations on human beings have been successful for the past twenty-five years. The operation is performed to treat scars on the cornea following bacterial or viral ulceration, *keratoconus* (an abnormally curved, but clear cornea) (Figure 17) or trachoma. Unfortunately, in the countries where trachoma is endemic, there are often religious and social obstacles to the transplanting of the cornea.

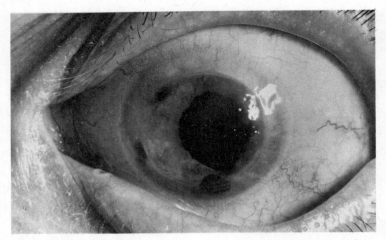

Figure 18 Corneal graft

Donor material may come from any adult, no matter what the cause of death, provided it was not an infectious disease. The eye (Figure 18) must be removed within 8 hours of death and used within 48 hours. The National Eye Bank at East Grinstead makes a number of eye donations. The donor cornea is sutured into the host by fine, perlon sutures, preferably with the aid of a microscope. The sutures are so fine that they cause little irritation, and are removed after three months. Approximately 70 per cent of corneal grafts are successful.

Rejection can occur, but it is much rarer than in heart or renal transplants. This is because anti-rejection therapy, such as *cortisone*, can be administered topically in the eye. The antibodies which cause rejection are brought to the grafted organ by blood vessels, and fortunately, even in the most diseased cornea, blood vessels are rare. The worst prognosis obtains in chemical burns of the cornea, such as lime burns and ammonia burns.

Nursing care
The patient is nursed flat in bed for 48 hours after the operation. He is then gradually mobilized, since there are dangers in keeping patients in bed for too long, such as the risk of deep venous thrombosis. Antibiotic and steroid drops are instilled for two and a half weeks, and the eye is padded during this period. Patients leave the hospital with dark glasses, since they may suffer from photophobia. The newer type of sutures cause little irritation, and are usually removed three months after the operation.

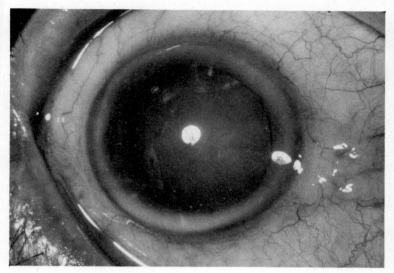

Figure 19 Cataract of the right eye

Cataract

This disease, together with glaucoma, accounts for 45 per cent of the blindness in the Western world. However, in Africa and the Middle East, trachoma is probably a more important cause of blindness. There is no reason why cataract should figure so prominently in the causes of blindness, since cataract operations have been performed successfully for the last one hundred and fifty years. Much research is still needed on the fundamental causes of cataract, but the main obstacles seem to be the difficulty in persuading patients to consult eye surgeons and the inadequate facilities in certain areas.

Cataract is a clouding of the lens (Figure 19). In most cases, the cause is unknown and, since it commonly occurs in patients over sixty years of age, it is referred to as a *senile cataract*, and considered in the same way as other senile degenerative changes such as greying of the hair and loss of skin elasticity. Inadequate diet and exposure to sunlight probably account for the high incidence of cataract in India. Of the rare forms of cataract, radiation is a well-known cause. It occurred in the people exposed to atomic radiation in Hiroshima and has also been found in hospitals where rays are administered for malignant conditions of the eyelids, when a lead contact-lens shell has not been used to protect the crystalline lens of the eye.

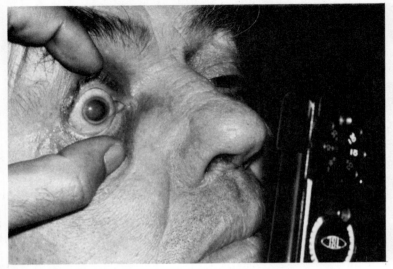

Figure 20 Diagnosis of cataract using an ophthalmoscope

The only symptom of cataract is a gradual failure of vision, and the degree of disability varies with the occupation of the patient. If he is a farm worker, the cataract may be well advanced before he is aware that anything is amiss but, should he work in precision engineering, he is likely to complain of deterioration of vision in the early stages of cataract. One of the more subtle effects of cataract is a defect in colour vision. It is now thought that Constable had cataract, because of the excess of brown in his later paintings.

The diagnosis is obtained by shining a bright light from an ophthalmoscope on to the patient's pupil (Figure 20), when the black cataract will be seen as a silhouette against the red reflex of the retina. It can also be examined with the slit–lamp microscope.

Treatment
An indication that an operation is necessary is if the patient has eyesight difficulty in carrying out his normal activities. A measurement of visual acuity indicating the need for operation is 6/18 (this corresponds to the fourth line on the standard chart when the patient is standing 6 metres away from it).

Because of the fears of many patients, a variety of pseudo-cures have always been available, and some are still advertised today. However, there have been rapid advances in surgical treatment within the past ten years. This may be carried out under general or local anaesthesia. General anaesthesia is preferable, especially if the anaesthetist is expert, since the patient must not vomit or cough in the post-operative period, or the delicately sutured wound may break. However, local anaesthesia, although less satisfactory, is still used in many cases. The surface of the patient's eye is anaesthetized with cocaine drops and he is given an injection into the orbit to affect the nerves sustaining pain within the eye. Squeezing of the eyelids during the operation would be disastrous, so the facial nerve is blocked by an injection just in front of the lobe of the ear.

The patient must be relaxed and apathetic during this procedure, so that drugs such as *pethedine* (75 mg), *sparine* (50 mg) or *phenergan* (25 mg) are commonly given an hour before the operation.

The operation (Figure 21) involves making an incision around half the circumference of the cornea. The lens is grasped by a fine forceps attached to the capsule or envelope, or a frozen probe may be stuck on to the surface of the lens. The corneal wound is sutured with very fine silk or nylon.

Post-operative care
Patients are allowed to get out of bed on the day after the operation and may sit in an armchair. This reduces the risk of deep venous thrombosis. They should be warned not to bend or stoop, as this causes a rise in pressure in the neck veins, which in turn increases the pressure in the eye and may rupture the delicate wound. Although patients like to be independent, they should be protected from injuring themselves, so should not be allowed to lean out of bed in case they knock the operated eye. However, it is probably better to allow them to walk (accompanied) to the lavatory rather than to give them bedpans. If the nursing is inadequately supervised, the patient may suffer *hyphaema* (bleeding into the anterior chamber), rupture of the wound or infection.

Most patients leave hospital about one week after the operation. Older patients should be carefully supervised to ensure that there is someone, such as a relative, who can instil the necessary drops (*atropine* and an antibiotic), and also that they will not have to do their own cooking, because visual improvement takes some weeks and there is the risk of accidents occurring.

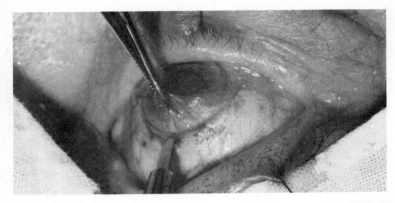

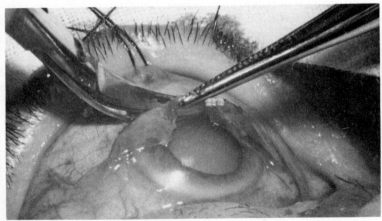

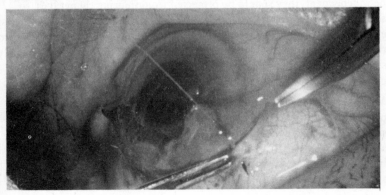

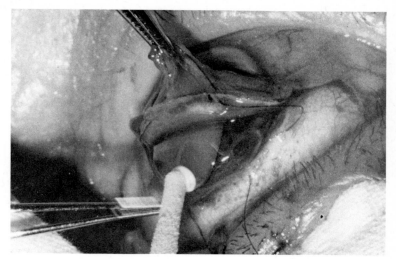

Figure 21 The operation for cataract.
1 An incision is made at the corneo–scleral junction (*limbus*) using a simple razor; note that the conjunctiva is reflected forwards and held by forceps; 2 The incision is enlarged by scissors; 3 A fine suture is inserted at the corneo–scleral junction; 4 The cataractous lens is being withdrawn by a cold probe, which sticks to the lens

To achieve the maximum benefit from the operation, the patient should wear special cataract spectacles. These must be prescribed six weeks after the operation, but the hospital will often lend the patient a temporary pair of spectacles which will enable him to get about and perhaps watch television, although he will not be able to read.

Cataracts in children

These are often familial but are sometimes due to German measles (*rubella*) contracted by the mother during the first eight weeks of pregnancy. The operation must be performed within the first few months after birth so that the macula can develop. A different operating technique is involved from that described above for senile cataract, since the lens in the eye of the infant is soft and can be sucked out with a needle and syringe. After the operation, the child must wear heavy cataract glasses, or sometimes contact lenses, in order to see.

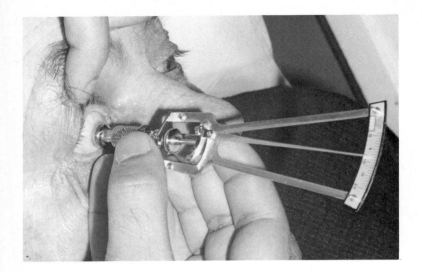

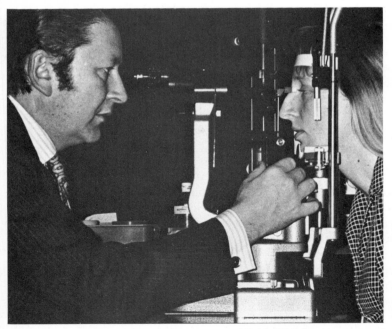

Figure 22 Checking the intraocular pressure with (*a*) Shiotz's tonometer and (*b*) an applanation tonometer

Chronic glaucoma

This disease, with cataract, is responsible for a great deal of the blindness in the world. The condition involves a rise in the intraocular pressure and the main disability it causes is a defect in the visual field, the area the patient can see around him. It is quite different from *acute glaucoma* (see p. 32).

The intraocular pressure is normally 20 mmHg (millimetres of mercury), and is measured with a special instrument, a *tonometer* (Figure 22), which is placed on the anaesthetized eye. The change brought about by the raised intraocular pressure is insidious and takes place over many months so that the average patient does not realize he is gradually becoming blind. Over the months, the retinal receptors are damaged by the raised pressure and the fibres of the optic nerve (the nerve has about a million fibres) gradually die. The patient commonly discovers he is suffering from this disease when he closes one eye accidentally and discovers that the other eye is almost blind.

It is important that this disease should be diagnosed in its early stages. The trained oculist, whenever he performs a routine test for spectacles, always checks the intraocular pressure, and also examines the optic disc with the ophthalmoscope for evidence of atrophy or the death of nerve

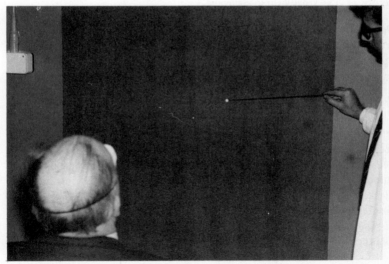

Figure 23 Checking the visual field – checking the patient's side vision

fibres. If the optic disc is cupped, glaucoma is established. The patient's side vision is checked, with an instrument known as a perimeter (Figure 23). If some of the patient's visual field is found to be missing (Figure 24), or if he has a blind spot (*scotoma*), glaucoma is present.

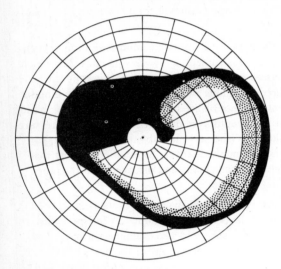

Figure 24 The visual field in glaucoma

Despite intensive research, the basic cause of glaucoma is not known. It is probably a result of an obstruction in the canal of Schlemm which drains aqueous humour into the veins of the eye. Some cases are familial, and a few are caused by doctors incorrectly prescribing cortisone drops.

Treatment
The intraocular pressure can be reduced by instilling drops of *pilocarpine* or *eserine* three or four times daily, and these constrict the pupil. If such drugs are inadequate, they may be supplemented by tablets of *diamox*, a weak diuretic which has a specific effect on the secretion of aqueous humour. The patient's intraocular pressure and visual fields must be checked at three-monthly intervals. If medical treatment fails to control the glaucoma, a surgical operation must be carried out in which an artificial passage is formed for the drainage of the aqueous humour under the conjunctiva.

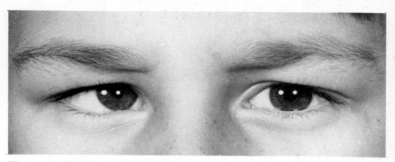

Figure 25 Convergent squint of the right eye

Squint (strabismus)

Normally, the axes of the eyes are parallel although, when a close object is viewed, both eyes converge inwards. However, if one eye deviates inwards or outwards, the patient is said to have a *convergent* or a *divergent* strabismus or squint. A convergent squint (Figure 25) is much more common than a divergent one, and an upturning or a downturning eye is rare. If the deviation is gross, the squint is obvious, but small degrees of squint may need special tests to pick them up.

The simplest of these tests consists in observing the position of reflection in the pupil of a light source. For a patient with a left convergent squint (the left eye is turned inwards), the light reflex is in the centre of the right pupil, but is displaced outwards in the left.

There are two types of squint. *Paralytic squint* may occur at any age, but is more common in adults. *Concomitant squint* rarely develops after the age of three.

Paralytic squint

The cardinal symptom of a paralytic squint is *diplopia* (double vision). It may be due to several causes:

1 Damage to the nucleus of a cranial nerve, e.g. haemorrhage in the region of the third cranial nerve;

2 Pressure on a nerve by an expanding tumour, e.g. stretching of the sixth nerve by an aneurysm;

3 Injury to the ocular muscles in a head injury, e.g. trapping of the inferior rectus muscle when the floor of the orbit is fractured (Figure 26).

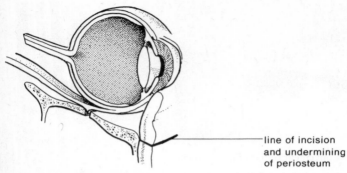

line of incision
and undermining
of periosteum

Figure 26 Fracture of the floor of the orbit, trapping the inferior rectus muscle

The symptom of diplopia is most marked when the patient is asked to look into the field of vision for which action of the defective muscle is needed.

A typical example of a paralytic squint is that of a thirty-year-old woman who was involved in a minor traffic accident because she momentarily saw two cars while parking. Later, when being examined by her doctor who had a pencil in his hand, she commented that she saw one pencil when looking straight ahead but, on looking to the left, she noted two pencils side by side. Her doctor found a left convergent squint using the test described on page 45, and deduced that she had a sixth-cranial-nerve palsy because the left lateral rectus was paralysed and the left eye could not be moved beyond the mid-line. On questioning, the patient admitted that five years previously she had weakness of her arm and leg. She was given a complete physical examination and an X-ray of the skull but nothing abnormal was found. A provisional diagnosis of disseminated sclerosis was made, and the double vision cleared completely after four weeks.

Concomitant squint

This is the squint of childhood. Although one eye may be convergent, there is no actual limitation of movement. The eyes are normally kept parallel by a conditioned reflex, which is acquired with difficulty in the first few years of life. As with any acquired reflex, it may be upset by an obstacle whether this be in the retina, the muscles, the brain or in the cranial nerves supplying the eye muscles.

Although the basic cause of concomitant squint is not clear, there seem to be two important factors. Firstly, 20 per cent of all cases have a family history of the disorder. Secondly, it may be a result of *hypermetropia* (long-sightedness) or the need for glasses to view near objects. Normally, in viewing a close object, we have to *accommodate* (make the lenses of the eyes more convex) and also *converge* our eyes. A two year old with long sight who becomes interested in pictures, for example, may accommodate excessively because of his long sight and he may also over-converge his eyes and develop a convergent squint.

An important difference between the concomitant squint of childhood and the paralytic squint of the adult with a head injury is that the child does not complain of double vision because the brain suppresses the image of the squinting eye. Unless appropriate measures are taken, this squinting eye will become blind. This defect is sometimes called 'lazy eye', but that is an inappropriate term.

Treatment of concomitant squint
Permanent poor sight (*amblyopia*) can be prevented by forcing the child to use the squinting eye. The earlier this is done the better, for it is usually too late after the age of seven. The first step is to test for glasses (*refraction*). It is simpler than might be imagined to test a child of two for glasses by objective methods. The baby's pupil is dilated and his accommodation paralysed by drops of *atropine* or ointment. These must be started three days before the test.

If glasses are necessary, they are worn during the waking hours and may need to be tied on. Many squints may be cured by glasses alone if they are prescribed at a sufficiently early age. Unfortunately, early treatment is uncommon because of the widespread but mistaken notion that squints will disappear spontaneously.

General treatment of squints
An important measure in restoring the defective vision of the spuinting eye is to cover the good eye (*occlusion*), usually for three months (Figure 27). Visual exercises can encourage the development of stereoscopic vision and help to keep the eyes straight after the vision has been made equal by occlusion, but these are usually not possible before the age of four.

If the squint has been neglected, an operation may be necessary for cosmetic reasons after the squinting eye has been improved by spectacles and occlusion.

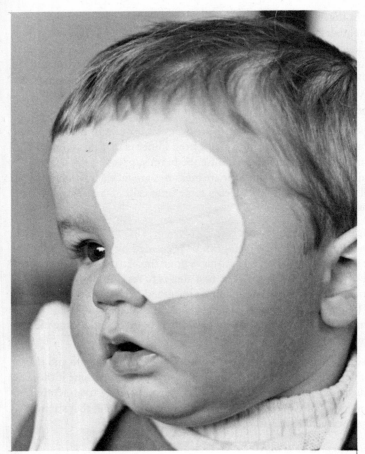

Figure 27 Occlusion

Watering eye (epiphora)

Tears are secreted by the lacrimal gland and drain into tiny channels (*canaliculi*) in the upper and lower eyelids. From here they go into the lacrimal sac and then via the nasolacrimal duct into the nose. In most cases the watering eye is due to an obstruction in the lacrimal sac or the nasolacrimal duct.

It occurs in two age groups, babies and the patient of fifty to sixty. In the case of the baby the obstruction is due to congenital remnants at the lower

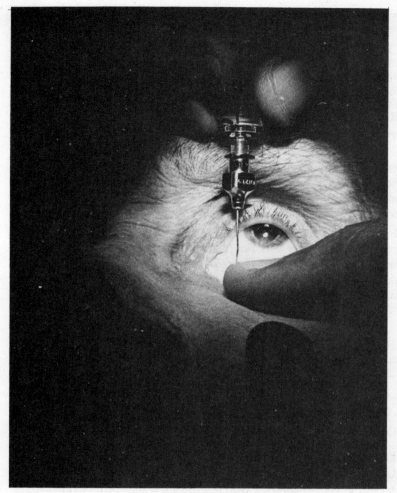

Figure 28 Syringing the lacrimal sacs, insertion of the cannula

end of the nasolacrimal duct. In most cases, the watering clears spontaneously by the age of six months but, if it does not, the duct can be probed under general anaesthetic.

For adults, the watering eye may be a cosmetic embarrassment and adversely affect the chances of their employment, for example, if they handle food, are dressmakers or climb scaffolding. Moreover, the constant watering may cause irritation of the lid margin resulting in *ectropion* (eversion of the lid margin). The treatment is to syringe or flush out the nasolacrimal duct (Figure 28), and this is successful in 75 per cent of patients. Where it fails, a short-circuit operation is performed, in which a hole is made in the side of the nose and the lacrimal sac drains directly into the nose (dacrocystorrhinostomy, D C R, operation).

Retinal detachment

This causes a gradual failure of vision. The patient commonly complains of a curtain ascending or descending in his field of vision. When the macula is involved, central vision is lost. Vitreous opacities presenting as floating spots in the field of vision or flashing lights are occasionally warning signs which should be taken very seriously. Many eyes with retinal detachment are large myopic eyes.

In the embryo, the retina is formed by the invagination of the optic vesicle, and the outer layer persists as the pigment epithelium. When retinal detachment occurs (Figure 29), there is a splitting through this potential space and the tear in the inner layer (containing the rods and cones) allows vitreous to seep in between the two layers.

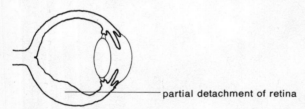

partial detachment of retina

Figure 29 Retinal detachment

Treatment
Until forty years ago there was no treatment, and the affected eye slowly became blind. Nowadays, retinal detachment is considered an ophthalmic emergency and the patient must be put to bed without delay. Strict rest in bed with both eyes covered for two or three days allows the retina to settle and the sub-retinal fluid to absorb. This is followed by an operation, of which there are several kinds.

In *diathermy*, an electrode placed on the sclera causes a sticky exudate from the underlying choroid so that the retina and choroid adhere. *Cryotherapy* has been one of the advances of recent years. A cold probe ($-70\,°C$ approx) is applied to the choroid and a similar type of exudate

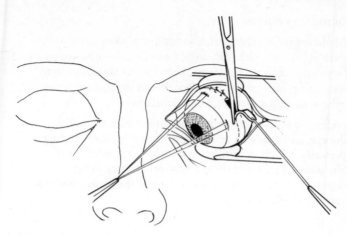

Figure 30 Scleral resection

sticks to the retina. In *scleral resection* (Figure 30), the eye is made smaller by removing a band of sclera. Another method is to tie silicone strings around the eye so that the sclera and the choroid protrude inwards (in the same way that a ridge protrudes inwards when a string is tied around a soft football tube). This then attaches to the retina. Approximately 85 per cent of all retinal detachment operations are successful.

Removal of an eye

Even if an eye is unsightly and blind, the surgeon hesitates to remove it because even a shrunken globe can be an excellent base for a cosmetic contact lens. An eye is removed for three reasons:

1 If there is an underlying tumour;

2 If it is blind and painful;

3 If there is danger of sympathetic ophthalmia. The cause of this is not known, but it is now considered to be an auto-immune disease, i.e. the patient is sensitized to his own tissues. It is well known that if there is damage to a patient's uveal tract from, say, a penetrating injury, the other eye occasionally develops a sympathetic inflammation. Early removal of such a damaged eye prevents the onset of this condition.

Summary of nursing points

The nurse should appreciate the particular nursing aspects in relation to the nursing care of patients with pathological conditions of the eye which include conjunctivitis, cataract, glaucoma, keratitis and their treatment. Her role is supportive, in regard to the physical and psychological care of the patient, who is usually under great emotional stress.

She must develop the skills of observing any patient with disease or disorder of the eye, and acquire a level of proficiency in administering any medication prescribed, such as instillation of drops or application of ointments. She must also acquire the essential proficiency in the pre-operative preparation and post-operative care of the patient undergoing surgery for cataract or glaucoma.

Chapter 3

The eye in systemic disease

The manifestations in the eye of systemic disease form an important aspect of diagnosis and help our understanding of certain pathological processes. Changes in the eye can readily be seen with the naked eye or with the ophthalmoscope so they can provide the first evidence of systemic disease. For the same reason, they are useful for checking the results of treatment.

Occasionally such eye signs may provide the only clue in a complicated diagnosis. They are of great importance in four common diseases: diabetes, hypertension, brain tumours and thyrotoxicosis; but here we shall deal with them on an anatomical basis.

The eyelids

Drooping of the eyelids is called *ptosis* (Figure 31). It may be present at birth or it may arise in later life from injury or disease. In early life, ptosis may affect vision if the pupil is partly covered, and such children often walk with their heads extended, sometimes being the object of teasing by their schoolfriends. For cosmetic reasons congenital ptosis should be corrected before school age by shortening the muscle of the eyelid (the *levator palpebrae*).

Myasthenia gravis is a disease in which patients first complain that their eyelids droop in the evenings and later that ptosis is constant. The cause of

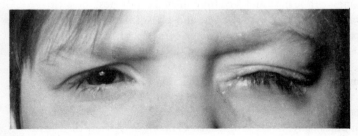

Figure 31 Congenital ptosis

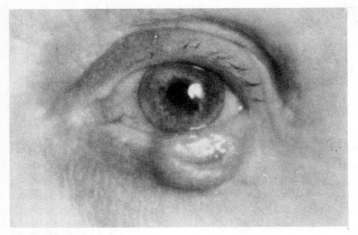

Figure 32 Rodent ulcer

the disease is not known precisely but it is probably a lack of acetyl choline at the nerve–muscle junctions. Women of middle age are more commonly afflicted. If the condition is not recognized and treated, other muscles become affected so that the patient may have generalized weakness and find difficulty in eating and swallowing. The diagnosis is one of the most dramatic. The patient is given an injection of *tensilon* (10 mg) and in 60 seconds the ptosis disappears if it is due to myasthenia gravis.

Rodent ulcers of the eyelid (Figure 32) are common, particularly in Australia, possibly because of the intense sun. They are a very slow type of cancer and can be treated by radiotherapy or removed surgically.

The cornea and sclera

These may show changes associated with skin disease, such as *acne rosacea* (a blotchiness of the nose and face from dilated capillaries), or with *congenital syphilis*, where usually a 'ground-glass' interstitial keratitis (semi-opaque cornea) is present, so that a corneal graft may be necessary. However, the most important changes in the cornea occur with *rheumatoid arthritis*, when the condition is known as *Sjögren's syndrome*. In this condition, the lacrimal gland does not function, so the patient cannot produce tears. Thus the cornea becomes dry and loses its transparency and the patient complains of irritable eyes. Artificial tears should be instilled six to ten times daily. Some drugs, such as *chloroquine*, show their toxic effects early in the form of a brown pigment on the surface of the cornea.

The lens

This is embryologically derived from the ectoderm, so the lens would be expected to become opaque or a cataract to form in certain skin diseases such as the asthma–eczema syndrome. The ligament that holds the lens in position is of mesodermal origin and, when this is deficient, dislocation occurs. The condition is associated with long, spindle-shaped fingers, weak musculature and heart abnormalities.

The retinal vessels

These are part of the cerebral circulation, and certain deductions can be made about the health of the brain and of the blood vessels generally when the retina is viewed with the ophthalmoscope (Figure 33).

The retinal vessels, because of their size, are called *arterioles* and *venules*. The arterioles may show narrowing, irregularity, tortuosity or frank obstruction. The venules may show dilatation (often referred to as 'sausage-like') or pressure effects from the overlying sclerotic arteriole. These are commonly called AV pressure changes.

Both arterioles and venules may have haemorrhages emanating from their walls into the surrounding retina. Similarly, the diseased vessels may have a defective circulation so that parts of the retina may die, giving rise to white deposits, inappropriately called 'exudates'. Occasionally a shining

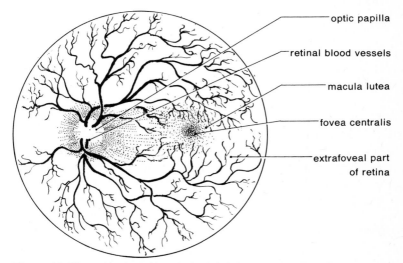

Figure 33 The retina seen through the ophthalmoscope

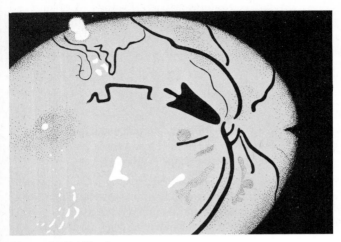

Figure 34 Papilloedema

crystal may be observed in the wall (lumen) of a retinal vessel, and this may give a clue to a disorder of cholesterol metabolism.

In *essential hypertension*, some or all of the above signs may be present. The haemorrhages and exudates usually disappear with the appropriate medical treatment (*aldomet* and *methyldopa*), but the hardened sclerotic vessels remain unchanged. In *malignant hypertension* (Figure 34) there is an added sign, *papilloedema* (swelling of the optic nerve). Malignant hypertension still carries a very serious prognosis for life expectancy, so no examination of the cardiovascular system is complete without an examination of the retinal vessels with the ophthalmoscope.

The eye changes in *diabetes* (Figure 35) arise about ten years after the diagnosis is made. They are not related to the severity of the disease nor to the method of treatment, but to the duration of the diabetes. Although diabetic cataracts occur, they are very rare and the major changes take place in the retinal vessels. The earliest change is the formation of micro-aneurysms (small balloon-like dilatations of the vessel wall). This may be the only change for five years, but it is eventually followed by small round haemorrhages which appear and disappear over a number of years. Yellowish exudates eventually occur. The exudates are not an inflammation, but are simply due to leakages from the vessel wall. These

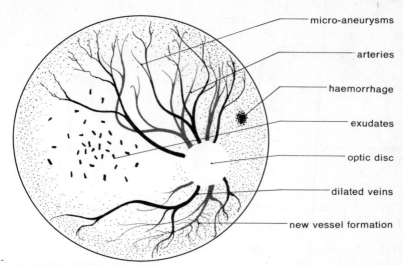

micro-aneurysms

arteries

haemorrhage

exudates

optic disc

dilated veins

new vessel formation

Figure 35 Retinal damage due to diabetes

cheese-like masses also grow and decrease over a number of years, while new retinal vessels may form. Eventually the haemorrhages persist and organize into fibrous tissue. When this fibrous tissue contracts, the retina is pulled away from the underlying choroid, and blindness ensues.

No satisfactory therapy is available at the moment for this *diabetic retinopathy*. Although proper control of the diabetes is generally desirable, it seems to have little effect on the development of the eye changes. New vessel formation can be temporarily stopped by the laser or light coagulator. In very advanced cases removal of the pituitary (*hypophysectomy*) is of some benefit, but the side-effects of this operation are serious so that it is not, at present, an accepted measure.

The optic nerve and tracts

The optic nerve is a collection of retinal nerve fibres which pursue a complicated course to the *occipital cortex* (the posterior part) of the brain. In the process the nerves divide, skirting the pituitary, and in this region they are frequently affected by expanding lesions, usually pituitary tumours (Figure 36).

If the optic nerve is compressed, blind spots (*scotomata*) affect the field of vision. Temporal field defects (i.e. the outer parts of the visual field are affected) may be the earliest signs of a pituitary tumour.

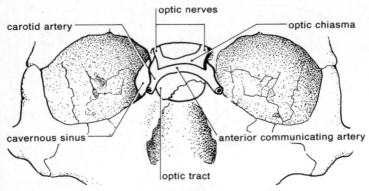

Figure 36 A pituitary tumour compressing the fibres of the optic tract (the cerebral hemispheres have been removed)

If the optic tracts are damaged, say by a haemorrhage in the internal capsule, half the visual field in each eye is affected. This is referred to as a left or right *homonymous hemianopia*. If such a patient is shown two pencils, one in front of each eye, he sees only one.

Disseminated sclerosis frequently affects the optic nerve so that it becomes atropic, causing visual-field defects and occasionally blindness of one eye.

Papilloedema is a swelling of the optic-nerve head (see Figure 34) caused by pressure within the optic-nerve sheath. In most cases it is due to a raised intracranial pressure, and is the classical as well as the most common manifestation of an *intracranial tumour*. The tumour may not necessarily be malignant and thus may occur in the relatively benign *meningioma*. Although brain tumours are an uncommon cause of headache, examination of the optic disc with an ophthalmoscope is essential in such patients.

Graves' disease (*thyrotoxic exophthalmos*) is a condition which arises particularly in women aged 20–50 years together with general signs of nervousness, tremor, sweating, loss of weight and tachycardia (increased heart rate). The patients have a characteristic wide-eyed stare with lid retraction, and a mild degree of protrusion of the eye (*exophthalmos*) occurs (Figure 37). This is due to pathological changes in the orbital fat. The exophthalmos is usually less marked than a first impression might imply, since it may be simulated by lid retraction. The eye changes are due to an excess of circulating thyroid hormone and may appear with a toxic

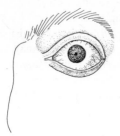

Figure 37 Lid retraction of thyrotoxic exophthalmos; note small pupil

thyroid adenoma of with the diffuse form of goitre. These eye signs resolve spontaneously in 95 per cent of cases when the condition is corrected medically or by thyroid surgery.

It is estimated that 1 per cent of thyroid patients develop *thyrotropic* or *endocrine exophthalmos* (Figure 38). Sometimes this develops after surgery and frequently the systemic signs of thyrotoxicosis are mild. It is, however, a serious eye condition. The patient complains of double vision, watering, and a gritty sensation. The eyes become progressively more prominent

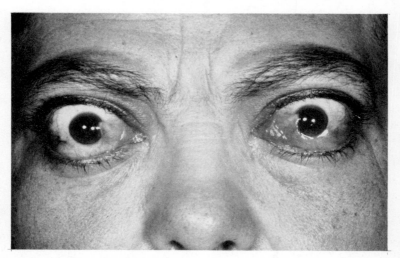

Figure 38 Thyrotropic exophthalmos

with redness and puffiness of the lids, there may be difficulty in closing the eyes, and ulcers may occur from exposure. There is no satisfactory treatment, but fortunately the condition is self-limiting and the active state lasts for only two or three years. During this period, the cornea must be protected by ointments when the patient is asleep. Occasionally it may be necessary to stitch the lateral margins of the lids together (*tarsorrhaphy*). In extreme cases, when the patient is quite unable to close his eyes, the tense orbital contents must be allowed to expand by removing part of the roof (*orbital decompression*).

Summary of nursing points

The nurse should appreciate the importance of the eye as an aid to diagnosis in diseases such as malignant hypertension, rheumatoid arthritis, disseminated sclerosis and intracranial tumour.

Part two

The ear, nose and throat

Author's preface

In writing a text book for nurses one must steer between Scylla and Charybdis – on the one hand avoiding a second-class text book for medical students and on the other hand not leaving out those details which are vitally important from the nurse's point of view.

Many of the diseases which afflict man assault him through the nose and throat and ears, and yet the study of those diseases and their diagnosis and treatment is relegated to a very short and often neglected part of a nurse's training.

In this book I have endeavoured to present in readable form some of the essential details of the conditions which afflict our patients in that region, together with some of the treatment, viewed as far as possible from the point of view of a nurse. I hope that this will assist my readers to understand a little about the conditions they are called upon to deal with and stimulate them to a further study of the speciality which is in fact far more important than it is often given credit for.

My thanks are due to all those friends and colleagues who have assisted and encouraged me in this project and the editorial staff of Penguin Education, whose expertise has made the preparation of the manuscript and illustrations such an enjoyable task.

H. Noël Waller

Chapter 4　　　The nose

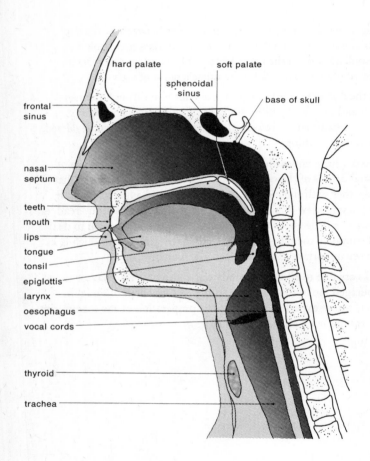

Figure 39 Vertical section through the skull and neck

The nose is the most prominent feature of the human face (Figure 39), projecting further forward than any other structure and receiving more injuries than any other organ in the body. Its shape varies in different races, and similar nose shapes are inherited by each generation from its predecessors. This extends to the internal structure of the nose as well as its exterior appearance, and deviations of the shapes of the nasal passages, as well as sinus troubles, can be passed on from one generation to another.

The anatomy of the nose

The nose is made up of a bony structure to which is attached a cartilaginous part. This cartilage maintains the shape of the nostrils and gives it the distinctive appearance. In infancy and during growth the cartilage is relatively soft and easily damaged, so deformity of the cartilaginous part of the nose is very common. The early foetal development of the nose is shown in Figure 40. The nasal bones develop from the nasal capsule in the mesenchyme (the layer which intervenes between the forebrain and the mouth), although the central bone of the nose (*the vomer*), which divides the two nostrils, is complete at birth. Projecting forward and making up the major part of the external nose are the hyaline cartilages of the nasal capsule. These never ossify, and become the septal and external cartilages of the nose, maintaining the external structure of the nostrils and about two-thirds of the bridge of the nose.

The nasal passages or nostrils are separated by a structure called the *nasal septum* (Figure 41). This is made up partly of cartilage and partly of bone, and may or may not lie in the midline (Figure 42). The opening of the nostrils leads into the *vestibules* (meaning 'entrance hall'). These are lined with squamous epithelium and contain sweat glands and hair follicles which, in older people, may produce a marked growth of hair in the nostrils. Infections of the vestibules are very common, and can be extremely painful.

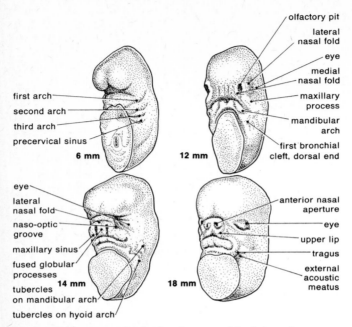

Figure 40 Four stages in the development of the human face

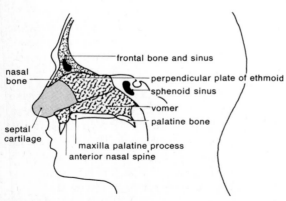

Figure 41 The nasal septum

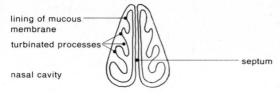

lining of mucous membrane

turbinated processes

nasal cavity

septum

Figure 42 Section of the nasal cavity

Deviations from the normal development of the nasal cartilages and trauma to them during their developing phase can result in the condition of *deviated nasal septum* (see p. 75), and may cause nasal obstruction, chronic sinus infection and nose bleeding later on. The condition of deviated nasal septum may often be traced to a comparatively minor accident in childhood. If a child has had a severe fall on the nose, even though there may not appear to be any displacement, the parents would be well advised to seek a medical opinion. The anterior nasal structures in infancy bend rather than snap, and the minor procedure of lifting the depressed anterior nasal structures may be very beneficial.

Functions of the nose

The nose has two main functions. Firstly, it is the organ concerned with breathing, providing a passage for the air to pass through during inhalation and expiration (Figure 43). During inhalation, the nostrils carry air from the outer atmosphere (where it may be cold or hot, dry or wet,

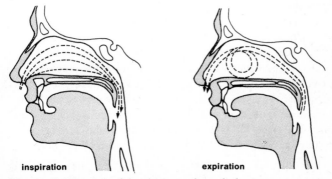

inspiration　　　　　expiration

Figure 43 The path of the airstream through the nose

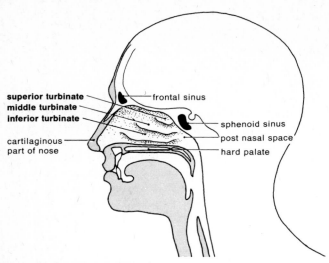

Figure 44 Lateral wall of the nose showing the turbinate bones

dusty, clear or containing noxious odours) down the nasopharynx (see p. 97) and through the larynx to the lungs. During its passage, the dust must be filtered out, the humidity corrected and temperature adjusted to one suitable for the specialized tissues of the lungs to receive it.

The healthy nose is able to carry out all these things remarkably successfully by means of the *mucous membrane*. The nasal passages are lined with columnar ciliated epithelium, which contains many secretory glands. There are also three very important bones in the lateral wall of the nose called *turbinates* or *conchae* (Figure 44). These are covered with ciliated epithelium, and the lowest and largest of them is the *inferior turbinate*. This is covered with erectile tissue lying under the mucosa which can be engorged with blood and increase its size almost instantaneously under the control of the autonomic nervous system. When the air enters the nose, it passes over the inferior turbinate and along the floor of the nose. The change of size and temperature of the inferior turbinate can therefore adapt the inhaled air for reception by the lungs.

Air is exhaled via a different course through the nose (see Figure 43), rolling down the upper part of the nose over the middle and superior turbinates.

A second function of the nose is to receive smells. There is a series of small holes in the roof of the nose where the lateral walls and the septum join (the *cribriform plate*). Through these holes pass the terminal fibres of the olfactory nerve. These terminal fibres are stimulated by odour which results in messages being sent to the olfactory centre of the brain which interprets them as smells and, to some extent, as taste (the two sensations are closely related). The sense of smell may be destroyed by central causes, such as virus infections of the nerve, encephalitis, influenza and intracranial abscesses and neoplasms, or by peripheral causes, such as trauma to the ethmoid sinuses resulting in the fracture of the cribriform plate or diseases of the ethmoid bones. Local spread of malignant disease may involve the cribriform plate, destroying the sense of smell.

The blood and nerve supply to the nose

Blood supply

The nose has an extensive blood supply (Figure 45) from the great arteries of the neck, the *common carotid arteries*. These leave the chest in the carotid sheath and divide at the level of the thyroid cartilage (Adam's

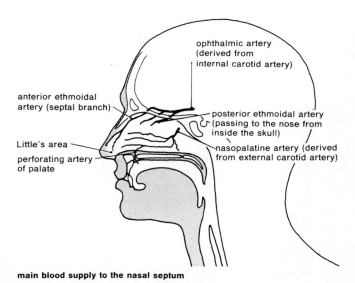

main blood supply to the nasal septum

Figure 45 The blood supply of the nose

apple) into the *external carotid artery* (sending branches to the neck, face and scalp) and the *internal carotid artery* (passing up into the skull to supply the intracranial structures giving off no branches in the neck). The internal carotid artery leads to the *ophthalmic artery* whose anterior and posterior ethmoidal branches supply the ethmoidal cells and the surrounding mucous membrane high up in the nose. These branches enter the nose from the orbit (and also supply the lateral part of the nose antero-superiorly), so bleeding in the back of the nose may come from these vessels.

The other sources of blood supply to the nose come from branches of the external carotid artery. The lower part of the back of the nose is supplied from branches of the palatine vessels, which come from the external carotid artery. Anterior branches of this artery supply the front of the septum and come up through the floor of the nose just behind the vestibule. The region where these vessels meet is called *Little's area* and is a frequent site for nose bleeding (*epistaxis*, see p. 78).

Nerve supply

The ordinary sensory nerves (Figure 46) are derived from the ophthalmic

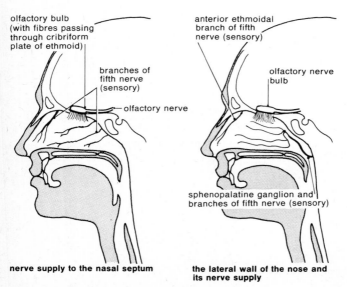

Figure 46 The nerve supply of the nose

and maxillary divisions of the fifth cranial nerve (the trigeminal nerve) and the motor nerves are derived from the seventh cranial nerve (facial). The sense of smell is governed by the olfactory nerve, described above. The dilatation and constriction of the mucous membrane and the turbinates is controlled by the autonomic nervous system, there being both sympathetic and parasympathetic fibres present.

The blood and nerve supply of the nose are closely associated, and those nerves which supply the mucous membrane of the nose also control the flow of blood through the plexus of vessels which lie under this membrane. Thus the mucous membrane can become engorged and swollen almost instantaneously. The amount of blood present and the degree of engorgement control the temperature of the inspired air, raising and lowering it as required during its passage through the nose.

The nerves also control the secretion of the mucous glands in the membrane. These produce a sticky lubricant (*mucus*) which keeps the membrane clean and collects fragments of dust and other particles which may be inhaled.

Congenital conditions of the nose

Although fewer congenital conditions will be seen in a general hospital than in a children's hospital or department, it is important that they should be recognized and their long-term significance appreciated.

Congenital syphilis

This occurs when the unborn child is infected with the *Treponema pallidum* organism by its mother during pregnancy. When it is born, a purulent discharge from the nostrils ('snuffles') is characteristically seen. This is due to destruction of the septal and nasal bones and if untreated leads to the 'saddleback' deformity seen in the congenital syphilitic (Figure 47). The nurse should report any suspicion of this condition to the doctor in charge. If the baby has running eyes, this may be produced by infection with gonorrhoea from the mother's genital passages during birth. It is possible that, if gonorrhoea is present, syphilis may be also.

The unsuspected presence of syphilis has been greatly reduced now that obstetric departments carry out the Kahn test and the Wassermann reaction on every mother's blood serum before the baby is born. Other tests which may also be carried out are the gonococcal fixation test (GCFT) for gonorrhoea and the PPR test.

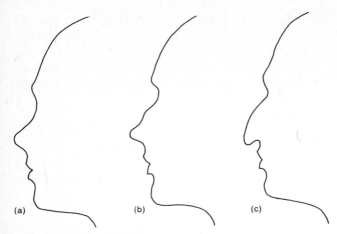

Figure 47 Deformities of the external nose.
The saddle nose of congenital syphilis (a) is due to loss of *bone*, whereas type (b) is due to loss of *cartilaginous* support, as occurs in Lupus or when the cartilage is damaged. Type (c) is typical of a post-operative or traumatic deformity

Trauma to the nose

The nose is the most prominent feature of the face and is particularly prone to trauma. Most children, at some time or other, fall on their noses. In infants and children, the cartilaginous structures of the nose are soft and pliable and do not easily snap, but they bend and can become dislodged. This can result in permanent nasal deformity, either twisting or depressing the tip, resulting in displacement or deviation of the nasal septum.

The bones of the nose may crack and bend producing deformity, or they may splay out, resulting in thickening of the nose. In adults, any fracture of the nasal bones can usually be seen and felt and will normally show up on an X-ray. If the ethmoid cells are fractured, a rim of bruising may be seen under the eyes.

Treatment
First-aid treatment is to bathe with ice-cold water to reduce the swelling and lessen the tendency to nose bleeding (*epistaxis*, see p. 78). It may be necessary to pack the nose with ribbon gauze soaked in liquid paraffin.

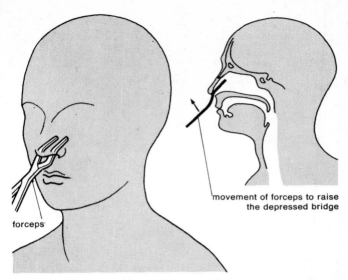

movement of forceps to raise
the depressed bridge

forceps

Figure 48 Treatment of nasal fracture while the patient is under endotracheal anaesthesia

Whenever any displacement is demonstrable, either in children or adults, reduction should be carried out under endotracheal anaesthesia (Figure 48). It is particularly important in children, where depression and thickening may occur associated with a deviation of the nasal septum which will probably become worse as time goes by, possibly requiring a submucous resection at a later date.

Sometimes a splint of plaster of Paris (Figure 49) may be used to immobilize the fragments in a bad break and the nurse should know when it should be removed and whether any packs present in the nose after the operation should be removed and at what stage.

The maxillary bone, ethmoidal bones and zygoma may be fractured in severe accidents such as road traffic accidents (Figures 50 and 51), and surgical intervention may be necessary. The depressed fragments are elevated and fixed in position either by dental splints in the mouth, or by special steel strut splints and a plaster skull cap (Figure 52).

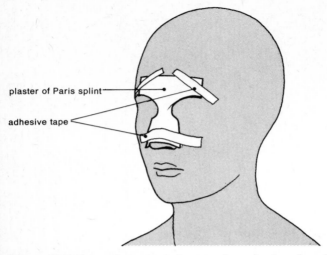

plaster of Paris splint

adhesive tape

Figure 49 Splint used to support the nose after reduction of nasal fracture

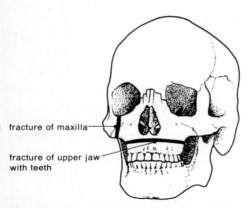

fracture of maxilla

fracture of upper jaw with teeth

Figure 50 Diagram of the skull showing fractures of the maxilla and face

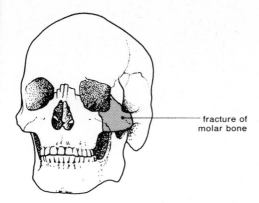

Figure 51 Diagram of the skull showing fracture of the malar bone

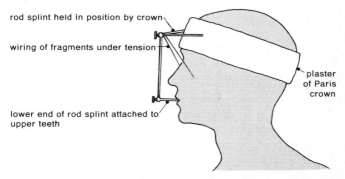

Figure 52 One method of retaining the depressed fragments in position

Deviated nasal septum

This is a very common condition (Figure 53) in the Western world. It may be the result of congenital distortion or it may be traumatic in origin. In the infant, the cartilaginous septum lies on top of the maxilla. It has its base in a groove running along the centre of the nose, with a ridge at either side. If a blow compresses the bridge of the nose, the base of the septum can spring out of position to one side or the other. When this first occurs, the deviation may be minimal but, as the child grows, the septum

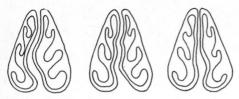

Figure 53 Types of deviated septum

also grows and the cartilage is pushed further sideways, causing an inferior obstruction. At the same time the cartilage may buckle in the opposite direction, causing a further obstruction superiorly. Thus, there may be an inferior deviation to the left and a superior displacement to the right. The bony part of the septum (the *vomerine plate*) may have been cracked, and this will also diminish the airway on both sides.

If the deviation is congenital, the inferior turbinates may often become enlarged on the concave side of the deviation as an attempt to equalize the airway between the two nostrils. This may result in a crooked appearance, though the patient may actually have little or no nasal obstruction.

Submucous resection of the nasal septum

This operation is designed to improve the nasal airway by straightening the nasal septum when it is deviated by trauma or is congenitally misshapen. Either half an hour before the operation, or in the anaesthetic room on arrival at the operating theatre, general premedication should be carried out. For example, *omnopon* and *scopolamine* may be given together with a local application of vasconstrictor to the nasal passages, either by spraying, packing or both. The usual solution employed is 10 per cent cocaine HCl in normal saline used on ribbon gauze. After spraying the nostrils once or twice, this is gently packed into the nose over the middle and inferior turbinates.

The operation consists of making an incision in the mucous membrane of the nose just behind the muco–cutaneous junction in the vestibule, and carefully peeling the mucosa and perichondrium off the septal cartilage over the whole extent of its irregularities. The cartilage is then split vertically, and the same process repeated on the other side. This leaves the irregular cartilage between the two layers of mucosa. The cartilage and any irregular spurs of bone are cut away and the mucosa allowed to fall

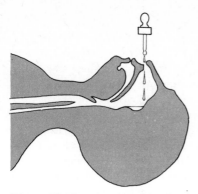

Figure 54 The correct position for the application of nose drops

together in the midline. The nose is then packed with supportive packing. Some surgeons use special splints, others use two fingers from a rubber glove packed with ribbon gauze, and some use tulle gras.

After the operation, when the anaesthetist judges that the patient has recovered sufficiently from the anaesthetic to return to the ward, the patient is wheeled there on a trolley, on which should be available a mouth gag, a wooden jaw lever, swabs, forceps and a kidney dish for vomit. The patient should be lying on his side so that secretion will more easily run out of the nose and mouth, and respiratory obstruction avoided. The patient's notes should be read by the nurse in charge, and any drugs given at operation recorded. The nurse should obtain instructions about the packing in the nose, its removal, and the steps to be taken if the patient removes the packing himself prematurely.

Forty-eight hours after the operation, the packing should be removed, taking care to remove first the pad in the nostril opposite the incision. Then the 'nose bag' should be replaced and ephedrine (0·5 per cent)/chlorbutol (0·5 per cent) drops in normal saline instilled into each nostril (Figure 54) three times a day to help keep the nasal airway clean. Sometimes tinct. benz. co. or menthol and eucalyptus inhalations may be given two or three times a day. The patient is usually discharged on the fifth day.

Foreign bodies in the nose

Most infants, at some time or another, insert unlikely objects into the nose. If not all the foreign body is removed by pulling or sneezing, a unilateral nasal blockage may result and, after a few days, there may be an offensive discharge. The nurse should not attempt to remove such objects, but should persuade the patient to seek medical advice. However, she should keep and show to the doctor all fragments which may come away. The only successful way to remove foreign bodies from the nostrils of infants is under general anaesthetic. The nose should be sprayed (using an all-glass atomizing spray) with a very small quantity of 2·5 per cent cocaine to reduce haemorrhage and give better exposure. Then, under a good light and using the appropriate instruments, the foreign body can be removed. There is no specific after care as far as nursing is concerned, other than to keep all fragments of foreign bodies. After the operation, the nurse should look after the child as it comes round from the anaesthetic, wipe its nose, and maintain a patent airway. Any fragments of foreign bodies which are sneezed up should be kept to show to the doctor.

Epistaxis

Nose bleeding (*epistaxis*) is one of the most common nasal conditions. The causes can range from nose picking or a blow on the nose, to local conditions like *vestibulitis* (an inflammation, generally with streptococci or staphylococci, involving the hairy part of the nose and causing ulceration and bleeding) or a deviation of the nasal septum causing excessive drying of the concave or obstructing part of the septum. If Little's area (see p. 70) is involved, anterior nasal bleeding is caused which comes from the vessels supplying that area. Common colds and sinusitis may cause epistaxis. In old people and in general diseases, such as leukaemia, diphtheria and hypertension, the bleeding may be posterior and is then much more severe, since the vessels involved may be much larger.

Treatment
First-aid treatment, which the nurse may need to administer, is to sit the patient up leaning over a sink and pinch the nostrils firmly together with thumb and forefinger at the edge of the nasal bones (Figure 55), for at least ten minutes. The patient should lean forward rather than lie down, and the blood should be allowed to fall out of the mouth into a towel. This is for two reasons. The first is so that he does not swallow his own blood, which might make him sick. The second is so that the doctor can see how much blood has been lost.

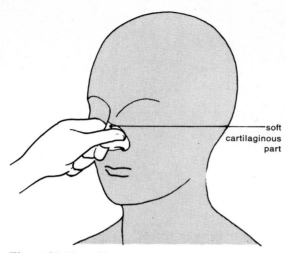

soft
cartilaginous
part

Figure 55 First-aid treatment for epistaxis.
Pressure exerted on both sides of the cartilaginous part of the nose will prevent
90 per cent of bleeding from the anterior part of the septum and nasal walls

A further intermediate measure which the nurse may embark on after
obtaining full instructions is to pack the nose with ribbon gauze (Figure 56)
moistened in *xylocaine* and *epinephrine* (1 part in 80 000) or liquid paraffin.
The packing should be inserted into the nostrils gently with the aid of a
pair of angular dressing forceps. Ideally, a nasal speculum and headlight
should be available to give good vision and exposure. The nurse should be
careful to watch for clots of blood, which may go down the back of the
nose and block the pharynx. Some cases may need to be cauterized. This
may be carried out in the out-patient's department. In children, it is often
sufficient to use silver nitrate as a cautery either in solution of
approximately 50 per cent strength, or else a bead of fine fused silver nitrate.
Alternatively, trichloracetic acid may be used. The anaesthetic in these
cases may be cocaine in a strength of up to 10 per cent, but it must be
used with caution. Children are happier lying down, but may be sat
upright if required.

The electric galvano cautery consists of a platinum loop through which an
electric current is passed via a transformer and a rheostat. It is possible to

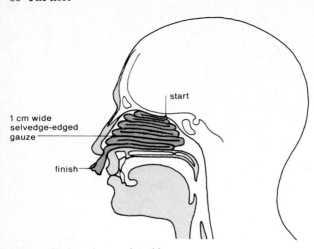

Figure 56 Anterior nasal packing

cauterize the mucosa very locally and deeply, but it is far more difficult to adequately anaesthetize the mucosa, particularly near the muco-cutaneous junction in the vestibule. The nurse should check that the appropriate solutions are available and that the transformer and rheostat are connected to the mains and working properly. It may be necessary to hold the patient's head while the procedure is being carried out. A few cases may need to be operated on for ligation of the anterior and posterior ethmoidal arteries or internal maxillary artery. Transfusion with packed cells may be advisable if loss of blood is severe.

When the situation reaches this stage, the nurse's part resolves into the realm of operative and post-operative nursing. In particular, the packing should not be removed by the patient whilst recovery from the anaesthetic is taking place, the blood pressure must not drop, and clots in the mouth and throat must not obstruct the airway.

Allergic rhinitis

This is a peculiar condition of inflammation of the nasal mucosa in which the mucous membrane of the septum and turbinates becomes pale and engorged, causing severe nasal obstruction, and pouring out vast quantities of serous fluid which pours down the nose causing considerable discomfort.

The most common type is *hay fever*, but there are many substances which can produce this condition, particularly the house-dust mite, pollens, and overstrong nasal drops and inhalants.

Treatment is complex, but desensitization with a course of injections can be successful. Various antihistamines produce symptomatic relief and long-acting steroids are currently popular, particularly in seasonal cases, since one injection may bring relief for the season. Sub-mucous diathermy of the turbinates is successful in intractable cases.

Nasal infections

The most common infection of the nose is the common cold, which is very infectious and can be serious in old people or those prone to chest infections.

Local infections of the nose are mainly caused by streptococcus, staphylococcus and the *Herpes simplex* virus. These attack the hairy vestibule and can cause furuncles (boils), painful ulcers and sores. One of the most serious conditions which can occur round the nose is a staphylococcal boil on the nose in the region of the upper part of cheek and root of the nose, or nostril, or upper lip. Venous drainage of this region is in connection with the veins which pass into the skull to the *cavernous sinus* (a large venous 'pool' which lies behind the eyes) and, if infection of the veins takes place and it spreads into this rather stagnant pool of blood, a lethal condition called *cavernous sinus thrombosis* (Figure 57) is produced which was almost invariably fatal before penicillin and antibiotics came into use. For this reason it is most unwise to squeeze a boil in this situation, as infection can spread through into the skull.

Nursing care of this condition consists of seeing that the patient is comfortable, administering the prescribed drugs with scrupulous accuracy, and obeying the instructions of the surgeon in charge. The latter will want to know any change in the patient's condition, any visual disturbances, vertigo or paralysis of arms or legs, any sudden rise in temperature and pulse, or other signs of deterioration in condition.

Erysipelas is an acute spreading surface infection of the skin which is sometimes taken for shingles (*Herpes zoster*). The skin is red, and bubbles appear on the surface, which is raised, hot and reddened. The nurse's part in the treatment of this condition is to see that the patient does not further infect himself by touching the affected area, and also that his utensils are kept separate and sterilized after use. Disposable utensils are coming into

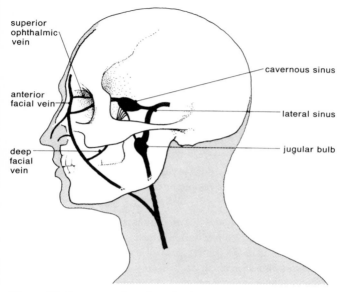

Figure 57 Cavernous sinus thrombosis.
The diagram shows the connections which facilitate the communication between the veins outside the skull and those inside the skull. Infection can easily be carried along these veins

more common use, particularly in hospitals. Barrier nursing is prescribed and *icthyol* masks may be applied to the affected area. Antibiotics such as penicillin and fucidin have a place in the treatment of this condition.

Herpes zoster can affect the nose, producing localized vesicular rashes which are often unilateral. It is a virus infection of the terminal branches of the fifth cranial nerve, so it is acutely painful and very potent analgesics may be required, as well as applying the drug Idoxuridine topically as a paint. Antibiotic cream can prevent secondary infection of the original viral lesions. *Herpes simplex* can also produce severe and recurrent lesions which tend to repeatedly develop at the same site.

Two other important local affections of the nose are *lupus* and *syphilis*. Lupus affects the cartilaginous part of the nose producing soft nodules which eventually break down to form ulcers. They heal with treatment, but produce considerable ptosis and deformity, particularly of the nasal tip (see Figure 49). Syphilis affects the bridge of the nose and produces the deformity of 'saddlebacked' nose (see p. 72).

Important structures in relation to the nose and sinuses

Above the nose lie the frontal lobes of the brain and the olfactory nerves, and behind and above the sphenoid sinus is the hypothalamus and pituitary fossa. Laterally the orbit is separated from the ethmoids by paper-thin bones which can become very soft and degenerated in the presence of infection, so that the orbital cavities may be damaged in operations upon the ethmoid. Below the upper jaw, the molars are in close proximity to the floor of the antrum, and their roots may even lie in the antral cavity. Accidental trauma or dental extraction can therefore tend to force teeth roots or fragments into the cavity of the antrum.

Dachryocystitis

This is an inflammation of the lacrimal sac, which lies below the eye and receives the tears as they drain away from the conjunctiva into the nose under the anterior part of the inferior turbinate via the nasolacrimal duct. The cause of the infection may be congenital stenosis of the nasolacrimal duct or it may arise as a result of chronic infection of the nose or lacrimal sac. Treatment may be by antibiotic eye drops and parenteral antibiotics but, in an intractable case, the sac may have to be drained directly into the nose by carrying out the operation of *dachryocysto rhinostomy*.

Summary of nursing points

The nurse should acquaint herself with the structure and functions of the nose. She should study such conditions as nasal infections and rhinitis and be aware of the principles of corrective surgery for deformities of the nose.

The nurse must become proficient in the skills required in caring for patients with nasal disorders and be aware of the importance of psychological care and support of the patient. She should acquaint herself with the preparation, care and management of any patient, particularly if it is a child, who is undergoing an investigation or test. Reassurance is vital to the successful outcome of such tests.

The nurse must also be conversant with the first aid that may be indicated in emergency situations, including epistaxis and nasal obstruction due to foreign bodies.

Chapter 5   The sinuses

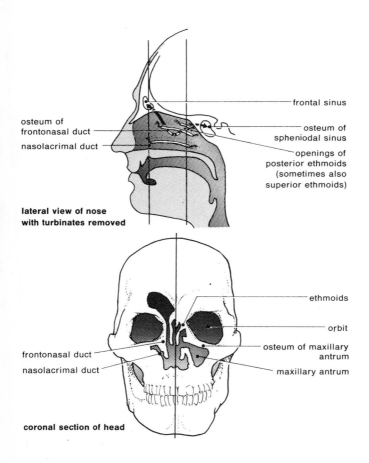

Figure 58 The openings of the sinuses and the nasolacrimal duct

The auxiliary nasal sinuses

A study of the human skull will show that there are a number of air spaces surrounding the nose and lying under the orbit of the eye in the cheek and also in the forehead. These air spaces are called the *auxiliary nasal sinuses* and consist of three paired groups: the *frontal*, *maxillary* and *ethmoidal sinuses*. The last are collections of very small air spaces, resembling a honeycomb and situated between the posterior part of the lateral wall of the nose and the orbit. They consist of three groups, the *anterior*, *middle* and *posterior ethmoidal cells*. The anterior and middle ethmoidal cells drain into the middle meatus under the middle turbinate, while the posterior ethmoidal cells drain into the superior meatus under the superior turbinate. The maxillary sinuses drain into the nose via the middle meatus under the middle turbinate.

There is another sinus, the *sphenoidal sinus* (see Figure 39) in the sphenoid bone lying under the pituitary fossa. It is not symmetrical and opens into the supreme meatus above the middle turbinates.

All these air spaces must open to the atmosphere to keep the pressure inside them the same as in the air outside. The pressure must obviously change as one climbs a mountain or goes down in a lift. This is achieved by the *osteum* (Figure 58) of the sinus.

At birth, the frontal sinuses are absent, appearing during the second year of life in the frontal bone and enlarging asymmetrically. The maxillary, ethmoidal and sphenoidal sinuses are rudimentary at birth and grow with the surrounding bone.

In the maxillary sinus (or *antrum*), the development of the second dentition of the upper jaw is liable to cause considerable irritation of the walls of the sinus, resulting in some degree of infection. After the upper second teeth have erupted, their roots, particularly those of the molars, lie very close to the walls of the antra. During dental extraction, fragments of bone or root may be forced into the antrum, or a fistula may be produced between the antrum and the oral cavity (an *antro-oral fistula*).

Diseases of the nasal sinuses

Any acute respiratory infection involving the nasal mucosa is liable to affect the sinuses. Normally, when the anatomy of the nose is sound and drainage adequate, the ciliary epithelium covering the walls of the sinuses and the turbinates will wash away the debris following infection, and the patient will recover. The common cold, for instance, goes through the phases of congestion and running nose, followed by resolution and thickening up of the secretions. These secretions then become purulent, are washed away and swallowed down the back of the nose.

However, if secondary bacterial infection has taken place and there is stasis and stagnation in one of the sinuses, a subacute infection occurs with swelling of the mucosa of the osteum resulting in the thick mucopus being trapped in the sinus. A rise in pressure then occurs, causing headache or facial tenderness and sometimes (depending on the virulence of the infection) swelling over the site of the sinus.

One of two things then happens. Either the pressure inside the sinus is able to force the pus through the osteum, or the sinus has to be drained by surgical procedures. The longer the infection is allowed to remain in the sinus, the more the ciliated mucous membrane deteriorates, even forming large gelatinous bags of so-called *polypoid mucosa* which may have to be removed.

Nursing care

The nursing of sinusitis is important. Good nursing in the early stages will stop an attack of sinusitis before the subacute condition has developed. The key to the cure of sinusitis is to keep the drainage going. Antibiotics are usually prescribed but, because of the poor blood supply of the walls of the sinus, the concentration reaching the organisms causing the infection is not very high. Decongestant tablets should not be used without specific instruction, nor should nasal drops unless prescribed by the doctor. The safest nasal drugs are Rx ephedrine HCl (0·5 per cent)/chlorbutol (0·5 per cent) in normal saline (100 per cent) used as nasal drops. Many of the stronger nasal drops paralyse the cilia in the nose. The body relies on these cilia to void the infected material, so these drops should not be used.

The patient should be kept in bed in a warm, moist atmosphere, obtained by placing a bowl of water in front of a fire, or on top of a central-heating

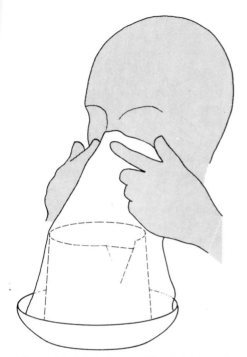

Figure 59 Inhalation, avoiding irritation of the eyes

radiator. The diet should be light with plenty of fluids, particularly hot, sweet, lemon juices. Hot flannels may be placed on the forehead and inhalations should be given. The Nelson's inhaler, although widely used, is not a very good apparatus, having too narrow a neck and producing vapour either too concentrated and hot, which is uncomfortable, or too weak when it cools off. It is preferable to make up the inhalation in a jug to the strength of 5 ml in a litre of just-boiling water, then place the jug in a fairly large bowl, wrapping a towel around the jug to make a 'gas mask', covering the mouth and nose (Figure 59). In this way the patient can inhale far hotter vapours than otherwise, since his eyes will be protected by the towel, and inhalation can be continued for about a quarter of an hour. Ephedrine drops may be given before and after the inhalation, which should be repeated three hourly. As an adjunct to these measures, heavy doses of wide-spectrum antibiotics may be administered and if a culture and sensitivity of the infecting organism becomes available the appropriate specific antibiotic can be substituted. Treatment with antibiotics should be continued for at least 14 days.

Surgical treatment
Surgical treatment of sinusitis may be carried out in the out-patients department under local anaesthetic, after which the patient may return home. The procedure is *antral puncture and lavage.*

Where conservative treatment has failed and after X-rays have been taken of the maxillary and frontal sinuses, the antral puncture and lavage is carried out to assist the drainage of the sinuses and restore the action of the mucous membrane to normal.

The anaesthetic is usually locally applied to the mucous membrane of the nose first by way of a spray of 2·5 per cent cocaine or xylocaine, and two or three puffs up each nostril produce a generalized minor degree of anaesthesia of the nasal mucosa. This then allows a probe, with some cotton wool attached, to be inserted into both nostrils beneath the inferior turbinates under vision using a headlight and nasal speculum. The cotton wool on the end of these probes is soaked in 10 per cent cocaine solution, or sometimes 25 per cent cocaine and adrenaline paste may be used. These probes should be left in place for at least fifteen minutes until no pain is produced by quite hard manipulations of the probes. The patient is more comfortable lying down, although some surgeons prefer to have the patient sitting up. Cocaine reactions are rare but can take place with a profound drop in blood pressure, pallor, sweating, very weak pulse, and even sudden death. More often than not, reactions are actually precipitated by fear of the operation to be carried out.

A trochar and cannula (Figure 60) are then inserted under the inferior turbinate and, about a centimetre behind its anterior border, the trochar is directed laterally and aimed at the patient's ear where the lobe joins the side of the head. With a gently rotating movement, the triangular point of the trochar is passed through the thin lateral wall of the nose into the antrum (Figure 61). The trochar is then withdrawn, leaving the cannula in place. A Higginson's syringe is then attached to the cannula and about one

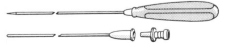

Figure 60 Lichtwitz antrum trochar and cannula

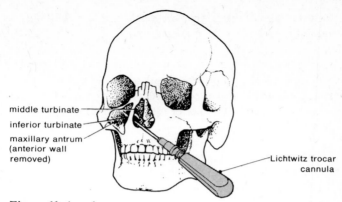

middle turbinate
inferior turbinate
maxillary antrum
(anterior wall
removed)

Lichtwitz trocar
cannula

Figure 61 Antral puncture.
The trochar and cannula enter beneath the inferior turbinate

pint of lotion made up of either sodium bicarbonate solution or normal saline at blood heat (37 °C) is washed through, with the patient's head hanging over a dish into which the lotion runs, carrying with it the fluid or semifluid contents of the antra – maybe pus, mucopus, or blood-stained mucopus. Swabs taken from the pus may establish the infecting organism and the appropriate antibiotic fluid injected and left in the antrum.

It is not true that, once a person's antrum has been washed out, it will continuously need to be washed out. Some types of nose are prone to sinus infections because of abnormalities and poor drainage and, in these cases, the correct treatment for an established subacute sinus infection is to establish drainage.

Antrostomy

If the drainage procedure is unsuccessful and the infection has become chronic, an *antrostomy* operation will be necessary.

Simple or intra-nasal antrostomy

Here, a permanent opening is made into the antrum through the lateral wall of the nose underneath the inferior turbinate. The surgeon can then remove polypi or degenerated mucosa from the inside wall and establish a permanent drainage, thereby allowing the infection contained in the antrum to subside. The advantages of this method are that it may be carried out either under general anaesthetic or, if necessary, under local anaesthetic. It is quick and usually effective. At the same time a bougie may be passed up the front nasal duct to enlarge it, and assist in the drainage of this cavity into the nose. A disadvantage of this method is that a full exposure of the maxillary antrum under vision cannot be carried out. Also, foreign bodies which may be lying in the antrum cannot be easily removed.

Radical or sub-labial antrostomy

This operation (the *Caldwell–Luc* operation) is carried out in cases where the infection in the antrum has reached such a degree that the mucosa is degenerated, and so much pus is present that an intra-nasal operation would be inadequate, since the inside of the antrum could not be visualized and infection of the ethmoidal cells could not be adequately dealt with.

An incision is made in the mouth at the junction of the buccal mucosa and the alveolar mucosa, and the periosteum is then retracted exposing the canine fossa which lies above the upper canine tooth (Figure 62). Here the wall of the antrum is usually thin and an aperture about 1·5 cm wide is

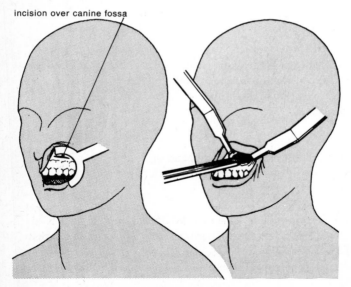

incision over canine fossa

Figure 62 The Caldwell–Luc operation

made in the anterior wall of the antrum exposing the contents of the antrum. Posteriorly, behind the antrum, the ethmoid labyrinth of cells can be seen. These are cleared of diseased bone, polypi and pus, and an opening is made (under vision this time) from the nose into the antrum. The cavity is then cleaned, including any ethmoidal disease. Sometimes, particularly if there has been a great deal of bleeding, the cavity is packed lightly with vaseline gauze, leaving an end coming from the antrum to the nose to facilitate removal, which can take place after 48 hours or, alternatively, a plastic drainage tube may be inserted to keep the artificial osteum open and left in place for three or four days. Irrigation of the antrum can be carried out through this tube post-operatively. The sublabial incision may be sutured with 00 catgut, but more often it is left without any suture, and heals up readily in a few days. Sometimes a foreign body, such as a tooth, may need to be removed at operation. Good clearance of ethmoidal infections can be made in these cases. Post-operative nursing is mainly concerned with oral hygiene. False teeth, if worn, should be replaced immediately after cleaning and rinsing out the mouth. A pad of cotton wool contained in a 'tubogauze' dressing should be fastened under the nose and looped over the ears to absorb blood and secretions which may leak out of the nostrils for the first few days (Figure 63). The packing

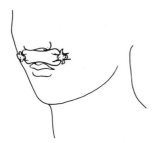

Figure 63 Nose pad of tubogauze with cotton wool inside

should be removed after 48 hours, or at the surgeon's discretion. It should be removed gently and smoothly, and if the patient is nervous, 100 mg of pethidene (or another analgesic) may be given to make the procedure less uncomfortable for him. After the packing has been removed, inhalations of vapour of tinct. benz. co., or menthol and benzoin, are given twice daily for the following four or five days and further irrigation of the antra can take place with a cannula at the surgeon's discretion.

Frontal and ethmoidal sinus infection

Although the maxillary sinus is the most frequently infected of the
paranasal sinuses, the frontal and ethmoidal sinuses can also become
infected. The frontal sinus lies behind the forehead and drains into the
anterior part of the middle meatus. When the maxillary sinus is infected,
this infection can track up the fronto-nasal duct and cause a *frontal sinusitis*.
Swelling of the mucosa occurs in the fronto-nasal duct, and pus and
infected mucus become trapped in the frontal sinus. As with any infection
confined in a bony cavity, the pus may break through the walls and
spread. It may spread outwards forming a subcutaneous abscess with some
infection (*osteomyelitis*) of the frontal bone, or it may spread posteriorly
into the cranial cavity forming an extradural abscess lying outside the
layers of the brain or even an abscess in the substance of the brain's
frontal lobe.

The ethmoidal cells can also become infected, usually in the presence of an
antral infection. This results in the whole labyrinth of the ethmoids
becoming filled with pus. Some external swelling can occur, since pressure
in the ethmoids rises. This swelling characteristically develops around the
root of the nose and orbit, as the ethmoid cells make up the medial and
inferior walls of the orbit. One of the most common results of chronic
ethmoidal infections is the production of *polypi* which swell up and block
the nasal passages. The walls of the ethmoid may even be eroded under
pressure to extend into the orbit.

Drainage of the maxillary antra by puncture and washout may allow the
infection in the ethmoids and fronto-nasal duct to be drained and subside,
thus reducing the swelling and the pressure in the ethmoids and in the
frontal sinus. However, if this procedure is unsuccessful, more radical
operative procedures may need to be carried out.

External, frontal sinus and ethmoidal sinus operations

These operations are carried out after failure of more conservative
measures, and consist of an approach via an incision under the upper and
medial part of the orbit and the side of the nose, to expose the fronto-nasal
duct and ethmoidal cells. Diseased bone, polypi and infected mucosa can
then be removed under direct vision. After the fronto-nasal duct has been
enlarged adequately, a skin graft is taken and inserted, with the raw side
outwards, wrapped round a soft plastic tube. One end of this tube lies
inside the frontal sinus, and the other in the middle meatus of the nose,

under the middle turbinate if it is still present. After ten to fourteen days, the tube is gently removed leaving the skin graft in place. Good drainage of the frontal sinus is obtained in this way. The external incision is sutured with fine plastic surgery silk, and it normally heals with a very cosmetic scar.

A nose pad (see Figure 63) is put into place and post-operative nursing consists of giving inhalations twice daily (see p. 87), and changing the nose pad as required. Alternate sutures are sometimes removed on the seventh day, and the rest on the ninth or tenth day, or earlier. A plastic dressing may be sprayed on, or elastoplast dressing applied if necessary.

Neoplasms of the nose and accessory sinuses

These occur in the region of the nose and among those occurring externally are rodent ulcers and epitheliomata. Some may be simple papillomata, while others are malignant and behave in a similar way to malignant skin conditions in other sites. They may occur in children and are often sarcomatous in origin. The nursing care is similar to that involved in the nursing of other malignant disease; in particular, strict aseptic precautions in dressing and post-operative attention. Treatment may be by radiotherapy or surgery, but the outlook is poor.

Carcinoma of the nose and antrum occurs in adults and, depending on the site involved, the treatment may be surgical, by radiotherapy or by a mixture of both.

Other general diseases which may produce ulceration inside the nose, with marked crusting and destruction of the tissues of the septum and turbinates, are collagen disease, sarcoidosis, malignant granuloma, Wegner's disease and leukaemia.

Nasal polypi

These are gelatinous growths which occur in the nose and are the result of changes in the mucous membrane producing bags of gelatinous tissue, which usually grow from the mucosa of the ethmoidal cells. Polypi may be formed as a result of chronic irritation due to allergic reactions, or they may be due to chronic infection and inflammation of the mucous membrane and disease of the underlying bone. They produce marked nasal obstruction and are often associated with hay fever or chronic sinusitis.

Polypi may be removed under local or general anaesthetic. A nasal snare is looped around the polypus and the loop tightened around the pedicle of the polypus. The polyp and its root are gently drawn down and completely removed, if possible. Sometimes when the polypi are small and multiple, forceps can be used to remove more localized polypi. In this out-patient's procedure, the nurse is responsible for holding a kidney dish under the patient's nose to catch the polypi and any blood, to wipe away blood and debris from the nostrils with swabs and generally to clean the patient at the end of the operation. A plug of cotton wool should be inserted into each nostril, to keep blood from dripping on to the patient's clothes. This procedure may also be carried out under general anaesthetic, particularly when the antra and the nasal mucosa are very infected, and in young children.

Summary of nursing points

The nurse should familiarize herself with the structure of the nasal sinuses and be aware of the real danger of cross-infection where disease or infection, such as sinusitis, is present.

She should be adept in the management of the patient following the operation of sub-labial antrostomy, and should be able to antrum washout, if required. As these conditions may affect children, the reassurance of the child, in lessening anxiety and fear, is of great importance.

The nurse should be conversant with the procedure of antral lavage, particularly the preparation and care of the patient, should these be indicated. When an inhalant is prescribed, the nurse should be capable of administering this; this may entail the use of the Nelson inhaler, as a medium of volatilizing certain inhalants such as tinct. benz. co. and menthol crystals.

Chapter 6   The mouth

Many important structures of the mouth and throat can be seen by looking into the open mouth. These structures are concerned with the first part of the digestive process. Digestion begins in the mouth. When the teeth crush the food to reduce it to a homogenous mass or bolus, the salivary glands secrete fluids into the mouth which not only act as lubricants but also contain enzymes such as amylase which help to digest carbohydrates. Looking into the open mouth, the papillae of the *salivary glands* can be seen in the floor of the mouth and on either side in the region of the upper second molar tooth.

The salivary glands

The salivary glands secrete salivary fluid into the mouth when the senses of touch, taste and smell are stimulated by food. The nervous impulses are conducted via the autonomic nervous system. They are reflex in type and not directly under conscious control.

There are three groups of salivary glands, the *parotid*, *submandibular* and *sublingual* glands (Figure 64). The parotid glands are situated on either side of the face, lying between the mandible and the mastoid process. If the parotid gland is inflamed (as a result of mumps, for instance), it is very painful to open the mouth, as the gland is squeezed between the muscle covering the mandible and the muscle covering the mastoid process. The gland contains three very important structures, the facial nerve with its five terminal branches, the posterior facial vein and the external carotid artery. Thus, if the gland is surgically removed, the operation is an extremely delicate one if facial paralysis is to be avoided. Each parotid gland has a *parotid duct* which opens into the mouth at the level of the second upper molar tooth.

The submandibular glands lie between the floor and roof of the submandibular fossa partly covered by the mandible and are each about the size of a walnut. The *submandibular duct* enters the floor of the mouth

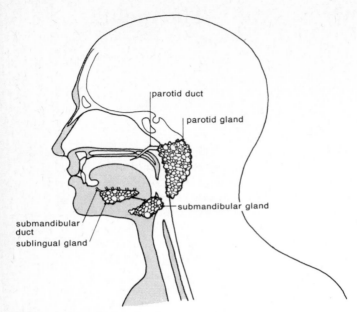

Figure 64 The salivary glands

on either side of the mid-line between the under surface of the tongue and the floor of the mouth. The ducts are close to the facial artery and the common facial vein.

The sublingual glands, situated in front of the submandibular glands, open into the floor of the mouth through numerous small ducts and produce mucus and enzymes to help produce the bolus of the food.

The tongue

The tongue is anatomically divided into three parts, an anterior two-thirds and a posterior third (Figure 65). The tongue develops from the floor of the embryological pharynx, the first and third arches forming respectively the anterior two-thirds and posterior third of the tongue. The anterior two-thirds are supplied by the mandibular division of the fifth cranial nerve (which is the nerve of the first branchial arch). This conveys ordinary sensations but, for the sense of taste, the anterior two-thirds of the tongue

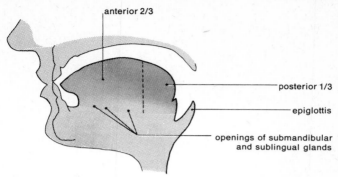

Figure 65 The tongue

rely upon the *chorda tympani* nerve which is derived from the second arch nerve. This second arch really takes no part in the structure of the tongue, for the third arch covers it over, forming the posterior third of the tongue. This portion is supplied by the glossopharyngeal nerve, which is the nerve of the third branchial arch.

Other structures of the mouth

On either side of the tongue can be seen two arches, the *palatoglossal arches* or *pillars of the fauces* which, at their lower end, join the base of the tongue and larynx. In the midline they are joined to form the *uvula* (Figure 66). Between these two structures lies a collection of lymphoid tissue called the *pharyngeal tonsils*. The palatoglossal arches separate the mouth from the pharynx and from the oropharyngeal isthmus.

Behind the base of the tongue can be seen the *epiglottis* which hangs over the pharynx and protects the larynx during the act of swallowing. Behind the nose and in the vault of the pharynx (the *nasopharynx*) are found in infants and children the *nasopharyngeal tonsils* or *adenoids*, which are masses of lymphoid tissue looking like a small walnut. These and the tonsils, coupled with the lymphoid tissue which is present on the base of the tongue posteriorly, make up *Waldeyer's ring of lymphoid tissue*, which can become inflamed in infection of the pharynx and nasopharynx.

The openings from the back of the nostrils into the nasopharynx are called the *posterior choanae*, and are usually symmetrical. Within the nasopharynx on either side are the apertures of the *Eustachian tubes* (see p. 128). These

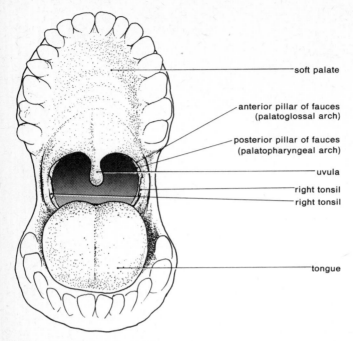

soft palate

anterior pillar of fauces
(palatoglossal arch)

posterior pillar of fauces
(palatopharyngeal arch)

uvula

right tonsil

right tonsil

tongue

Figure 66 General view of the mouth

are shielded by curved cartilaginous hoods with some muscular attachments covered by epithelium, and lead laterally and upwards to the anterior part of the middle ear. Normally the Eustachian tube remains closed but, if the pressure in the nasopharynx becomes raised (during swallowing, for example), the tube opens, allowing air from the nasopharynx to enter the middle ear and equalize the pressure. If this mechanism is disturbed, considerable pain may be experienced as the ear drum is compressed or distended.

The mucous membrane forming the nasopharynx is of the columnar ciliated type and is considered more as part of the nose than as part of the throat. Food does not normally enter this region since, during swallowing, the nasopharynx is shut off by the lifting of the palate. However, in certain diseases affecting the nervous control of the palate, e.g. diphtheria, *Herpes zoster*, anterior poliomyelitis, and sometimes glandular fever, fluids swallowed may be regurgitated uncontrollably down the nose, indicating the presence of palatal paresis.

The soft palate

This structure, which has a most important function in swallowing and breathing, can be thought of as a mobile posterior extension of the floor of the nose and the roof of the mouth. It is kept in position by the tension of two paired sets of muscles whose interaction can either raise or lower the palate as required. This action may be either conscious or reflex.

The *tensor palati* muscle tautens the palate and opens the Eustachian tube by pulling on the cartilage of the Eustachian cushion. This is the action which occurs in swallowing and equalizes the air pressure between the air in the middle ear and the air in the nose. The *levator palati* muscles form a sling which lifts the palate up when they contract. The posterior margin of the soft palate is then brought into contact with the posterior wall of the pharynx, separating the oropharynx from the nasopharynx, as occurs in swallowing. They are assisted by the *paravents* muscle, a U-shaped muscle which contracts horizontally like a sphincter muscle.

The palate is lowered by palatopharyngeus muscles which form part of the posterior pillar of the fauces. When contracted, these make the palate more arched and depress it to allow a free nasal airway. If they are not efficient in shutting off the nose from the pharynx, breathing through the mouth may occur.

Maldevelopments of the nose, face, lips and palate

During the development of the foetus, if certain ridges, tubes and septa do not unite in the later stages of gestation, anomalies and deficiencies can result. The most important conditions of this kind are *cleft palate* and *harelip*. There are many variations of these conditions (Figure 67) ranging from a double or *bifid* uvula to a complete bilateral cleft palate, with double harelip and complete deficiency of the floor of the nose (i.e. the roof of the mouth). The cause of these maldevelopments is generally thought to be some interference with the nutrition of the foetus or a toxic effect of a virus or chemical. A tragic example of this was the 'thalidomide' incident. If the disease German measles (*rubella*) is contracted by the mother in the first three months of pregnancy, it may result in congenital abnormalities in the child.

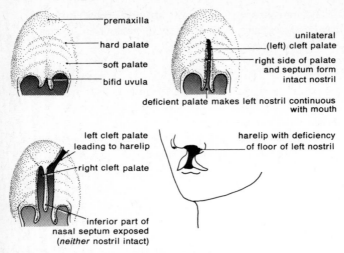

Figure 67 Forms of cleft palate and harelip

The importance of these congenital abnormalities and maldevelopments for the nurse is that deficiencies in the palate and the roof of the mouth and the lips make it difficult for the newly born child to breath easily, and normal suction is impossible for the child. Unless other methods of feeding can be instituted, adequate nourishment of the baby cannot be maintained, and its condition will rapidly deteriorate. It is therefore most important for the airway to be maintained. Sometimes a feeding tube passed through the mouth into the stomach may be used in the very early stages, but it is

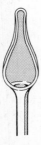

Figure 68 Spoon adapted for feeding an infant with a harelip or cleft palate

far better to feed an infant with a cleft palate or harelip by spoon feeding (Figure 68). With a little practice, it is quite possible for the infant to take its feeds in this manner, although the process is slower and more trouble than breast and bottle feeding. A disadvantage of bottle feeding is that, if a large teat opening is used, the baby is liable to be swamped by milk, and may choke.

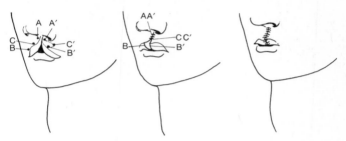

Figure 69 Mirault–Blair operation for harelip.
Incisions are made between A and A′, B and B′ and C and C′

Treatment of harelip
Harelip is usually operated on with plastic surgery at the age of three months (Figure 69). The baby should weigh 4·5–5·5 kg (10–12 lb) and should have a haemoglobin count of 10·5 mg per cent minimum. Before the operation, the nose and pharynx should be made sterile by swabbing for bacteria. If any infection is present, antibiotic treatment should be given. The operation is usually carried out under a penicillin cover.
After the operation, the baby's arms should be restrained so that it cannot touch its mouth. This is best achieved by keeping the baby in a carefully padded cruciform splint for the whole post-operative period, feeding the baby and changing nappies with the splint in place. It is only removed for bathing. It is important to check that the baby does not wet the splint, and that no chafing takes place around the back or arms. Care of the mouth and lips is very important. The first feed should be started about one hour after the baby recovers from the anaesthetic and, after every feed, four or five teaspoons of boiled water should be given to wash away any milky remains from the mouth. The lips should be kept dry and clean by mopping with cotton wool buds on orange sticks dipped in normal saline or spirit if necessary. Three to five days after the operation, the very fine nylon or silk threads approximating the suture lines are removed.

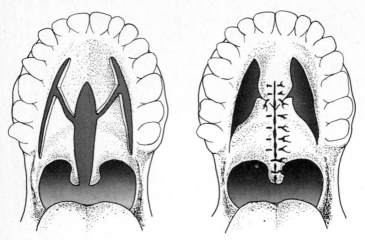

Figure 70 Operation to repair cleft palate

Treatment of cleft palate
This operation is carried out by plastic surgery (Figure 70), when the child is about twelve months old and before it starts to talk or the primary dentition has erupted. The same pre-operative care is carried out as for the operation for harelip (p. 101).

After the operation, since the baby is older, separate padded splints are used to prevent it interfering with its mouth. Feeds should be started one hour after the baby has recovered from the anaesthetic, with 225–250 g (7–8 oz) glucose water by spoonfuls, every four hours for 24 hours. In the second 24 hours, glucose thickened with baby cereal should be given every four hours. On the third day, normal homogenized diet can be resumed, but the feeds should be followed by several millilitres of boiled water, orange juice or Del Rosa syrup. For one month, no rusks or biscuits should be given.

In these operations, in contrast to those for harelip, the sutures are of catgut and so do not have to be removed. But the baby should not be allowed to play with sharp toys, pencils, etc., which may be forced into the mouth and damage the suture line. If food comes down the nose, it indicates that the suture line may have broken down producing a fistula between the mouth and nose. This is left for some time before re-suturing.

The nursing care of the mouth

The mouth and the *oropharynx* are open to the outside world, so they are more commonly infected than any other region, except the nose. For this reason and also because some patients, particularly old people and children, are lazy in dental and oral hygiene, the cleaning of the mouth should become part of the regular routine of looking after a patient. A clean mouth makes a great deal of difference to a patient's feelings and can give him a more cheerful outlook.

The natural teeth should be cleaned well with a soft toothbrush and toothpaste, although it should be remembered that older people's gums may not be used to this sort of attention and may be soft. Children should clean their teeth properly morning and night and, if they have recently had tonsils removed, they should also clean their teeth after every meal. Dentures should be cleaned with denture cleaner, then rinsed in weak disinfectant before being returned to the mouth.

If there are ulcers in the mouth, which can be painful, the doctor may advise that they be touched with a silver nitrate stick or possibly that a steroid tablet be placed over the ulcer and kept there until dissolved. A common infection in the mouth and on the tongue of babies and old people is *thrush* due to an organism allied to yeast. It produces characteristic white patches on the buccal margin, palate and tongue with a reddened and dry mucous membrane. The doctor should be told about the existence of this condition, when he may prescribe treatment with antifungal antibiotics such as fungilin or nystatin. A first-aid measure is to swab the mouth out, two or three times a day, with a solution of glycerine of borax or glycerine of thymol on a cotton wool swab attached to a pair of Spencer–Wells forceps.

Summary of nursing points

As well as understanding the structure and multiple functions of the mouth, the nurse must appreciate her own important role in caring for the patient's mouth. She must become thoroughly conversant with the pre- and post-operative care of the patient undergoing surgery of the mouth and be aware of the principles of corrective surgery for cleft palate and harelip (very often such patients will be young children).

Chapter 7   The throat

The muscles of the pharynx

The pharynx is made up of a tube lined with squamous stratified alimentary epithelium. It is surrounded by the *constrictor* muscles, which are paired structures inserted posteriorly in the mid-line into a medial fibrous vertical band called the *pharyngeal raphe*. There are three constrictor muscles, the lower ones lying outside the muscles above them (Figure 71). Between the base of the skull and the top of the *superior constrictor* there is no muscle in the nasopharynx, but fascia (the *pharyngo-basilar fascia*) through which, on either side, pass the Eustachian tubes.

The superior constrictor muscle is roughly circular in shape and passes backwards on either side of the mouth from along the mylohyoid line and

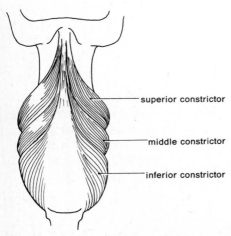

superior constrictor

middle constrictor

inferior constrictor

Figure 71 The constrictors of the pharynx from behind

along the side of the tongue. Posteriorly in the mid-line the muscular fibres fan out slightly upwards to the *basi occiput* and *median ligament* of the nasopharynx and downwards to the level of the vocal cords. Overlapping this muscle inferiorly is the *middle constrictor* which arises from the posterior edge of the stylo-hyoid ligament and the hyoid bone. The fibres of this muscle fan out to be inserted into the whole length of the pharyngeal raphe posteriorly. In its turn it is covered inferiorly by a portion of the *inferior constrictor*. This muscle is in two parts, the *thyropharyngeus* and *cricopharyngeus*. At its lower end it forms a sphincter (the *cricopharyngeal sphincter*), which shuts off the pharynx from the oesophagus. As well as being part of the pharyngeal muscle, this also relates to the oesophagus, being the end of the antechamber leading into the gastrointestinal tract.

The muscle originates from the oblique line of the lamina of the thyroid cartilage and also from the arch of the cricoid cartilage (Figure 72). The upper fibres wrap round the middle constrictor muscle and are inserted into the median raphe. However, there is a weak part at the lower end of the thyropharyngeus part of the muscle where the middle constrictor does not underlie it. Below this point, the cricopharyngeus is more powerful and passes in an uninterrupted semicircle of muscle without a median raphe joining the muscle of the upper end of the oesophagus. The weak area between the upper and lower part of this muscle is often the site of a *pharyngeal diverticulum.*

The motor nerves supplying the constrictor muscles of the pharynx, for the cricopharyngeus, come from the *nucleus ambiguus* in the brain-stem via the accessory nerve and the pharyngeal plexus. The cricopharyngeus nerve supply comes via the recurrent laryngeal nerve and the external laryngeal branch of the superior laryngeal nerve. The sensory nerve supply of the nasopharynx is derived from the *maxillary nerve* through the *sphenopalatine ganglion*. The oropharynx and valleculae are supplied by

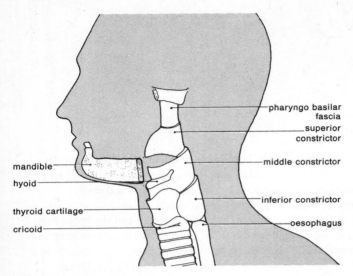

Figure 72 Lateral view of the pharynx

the glossopharyngeal nerve branches in the pharyngeal plexus. The vagus nerve supplies the laryngopharynx and pyriform fossa, via the internal and recurrent laryngeal nerves.

The blood supply of the pharynx comes from many branches of the external carotid artery.

The larynx

This structure is the gateway to the respiratory system and is also the organ concerned with speech. It is a complete structure made up of cartilage and membranes, surrounded by muscles and lined by mucous membrane.

The cricoid cartilage is the basis on which the larynx is constructed. This cartilage is the only complete ring in the respiratory tract. It has a narrow anterior arch and a deep posterior *lamina* and, near the junction of the arch and the lamina, on either side are joined the thyroid cartilages (Figure 73). Many muscles are also attached to these cartilages. There are other cartilages, the *arytenoid* cartilages, which are pyramidal in shape and

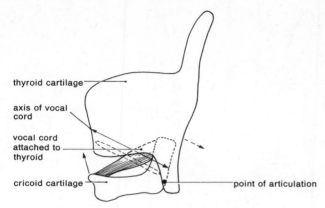

Figure 73 The larynx, thyroid and cricoid cartilages.
Contraction of the cricothyroid rotates the front of the cricoid cartilage on its
articulation with the thyroid cartilage in the direction shown by the arrow. This
stretches the vocal cords

which also articulate with the cricoid. These have both a rotating and
sliding movement, and are attached to the posterior end of the *vocal cords*,
being responsible for their movement (Figure 74).

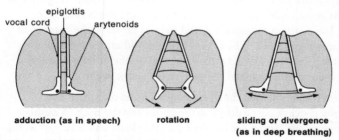

Figure 74 The arytenoid cartilages

The vocal cords are paired structures, lying side by side, and joined
together anteriorly in the antero-posterior plane to make up the *glottis*, the
opening between the laryngopharynx and the upper part of the respiratory
tract. During respiration, the vocal cords are slightly slackened and the

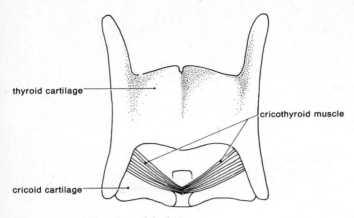

Figure 75 Anterior view of the larynx

laryngeal muscles draw the arytenoids apart, thereby widening the gap between the vocal cords and allowing the air to pass through the larynx.

When one starts to speak, the arytenoids rotate and are drawn together; in this way the vocal cords are tightened and, as the air is exhaled, sound is produced, which is then modified by the pharynx to produce speech.

The thyroid cartilages also articulate with the cricoid cartilage (Figure 75). They are the most visible part of the larynx, forming the *Adam's apple*. They meet anteriorly in the mid-line and help to preserve the patency of the entrance to the trachea. The cricoid and thyroid are joined anteriorly by a membrane, the *cricothyroid membrane*, and on the outer surface of these two cartilages are attached the external muscles of the larynx.

Above the thyroid is situated the *hyoid* bone. This is responsible for producing the concave curve dividing the chin from the neck. A number of the muscles of the larynx are inserted into this bone and take part in the act of swallowing. The cricoid serves as an anchor, remaining relatively still while the pretracheal and extrinsic laryngeal muscles contract, thereby raising the larynx.

Swallowing

Swallowing depends on the coordinated activity of the pharyngeal muscles, together with the muscles attached to the larynx and other structures of the pharynx, particularly the epiglottis. This allows food and fluids to pass

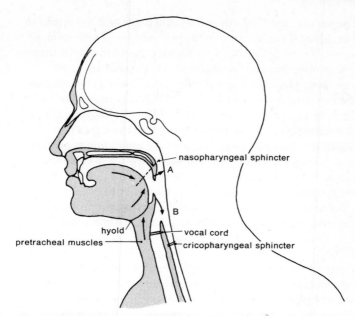

Figure 76 The movements of structures in swallowing.
The soft palate (A) rises to close off the nasopharynx. The epiglottis (B) moves to cover the larynx as the pretracheal muscles constrict and draw the larynx up with them. Beyond the nasopharyngeal sphincter, peristalsis takes place, automatically forcing food downwards. As the larynx is dragged upwards, the cricopharyngeal sphincter will be seen to relax and open

from the back of the tongue, past the entrance to the respiratory tract, safely into the oesophagus (or gullet) on their way to the stomach.

The food is prepared into a bolus by chewing and by the action of the salivary glands. The tongue then leads the food by contraction back to the oropharynx, where the reflex swallowing operations occur. At this point, the larynx draws up its opening under the shelter of the back of the tongue and the epiglottis, which tilts backwards. The glottic opening closes and respiration is suspended. At the same time, the soft palate is drawn up, separating the nasopharynx from the oropharynx. The upper, middle and inferior constrictor muscles then force the food downwards by means of a rhythmical movement called peristalsis (Figure 76).

Solid food passes over the epiglottis in a straight line whilst fluids tend to run on either side of the epiglottis into the pyriform fossae before entering the oesophagus. If there is disorder of swallowing due to structural changes (e.g. a neoplasm obstructing the hypopharynx) then solids are more difficult to swallow, whilst disorders of reflex action (such as neurological disease or neurosis) are more likely to produce difficulty in swallowing fluids, or fluids 'going down the wrong way'. When this happens, the laryngeal protective reflexes come into play and the larynx goes into spasm, bringing the vocal cords together violently and tightly to prevent further abuse. After a short time coughing will take place to expel any unwelcome materials from the trachea and bronchi. This is safe if the foreign body is small enough to pass into the trachea or to remain outside the larynx. But articles which can impact in the larynx may produce violent intraglottic spasm and eventually may result in asphyxiation.

General disease

The throat may be affected in many general diseases. One of the more important of these is anterior poliomyelitis, where paralysis of the soft palate, larynx and pharynx may occur. Progressive bulbar palsy, pseudo-bulbar palsy and polyneuritis can produce symptoms in the throat resulting in paralysis of the tongue and palate, and laryngeal paralysis affecting swallowing and making speech slurred. In leukaemia, lesions of the pharynx and mouth can occur, usually associated with ulceration and often bleeding of the gums.

The tongue may be considered a good indicator of the state of the stomach and the gastrointestinal tract. In acute appendicitis, a characteristic sign is a dry, furred tongue. The tongue may also appear dry and furred in other toxic conditions of the gastrointestinal system, in diabetes mellitus and in in uraemia. Alternatively, the tongue can become smooth, pink and sore in chronic anaemia and in certain vitamin deficiencies. Any infection or trauma of the tongue can be most painful, and carcinoma of the tongue is a particularly painful and distressing condition which should not go untreated or a painful ulcer will be produced and eventually the tissue may break down, leading to sloughing of the floor of the mouth.

Another condition which can produce severe symptoms in the mouth and throat, particularly in old people and in those who have previously suffered from rheumatism, is *Sjögren's syndrome*. In this condition, the secretions of the parotid submandibular, sublingual and nasolacrimal glands are either reduced or absent. This results in a dry sore throat, and reddened sore mucosa of the nose, oropharynx and mouth, causing considerable discomfort to the patient. Treatment with steroids gives some hope for patients suffering from this distressing disease.

Swallowing foreign bodies

Many children and infants accidentally swallow foreign bodies. If such a body passes beyond the oropharyngeal isthmus, it cannot return and, if small enough, will then pass by muscular contraction to the region of the larynx or cricopharyngeal sphincter. At this point one of two things will happen. It will either pass between the vocal cords into the larynx, where it may be checked by the violent reflex spasm of the vocal cords, or it may be inhaled into the trachea and main bronchi. The foreign body, depending on its shape and consistency, may be stopped at any point in this passage from the mouth to the oesophagus or lungs. The whole process takes only a few seconds, after which the situation is either immediately critical or else the emergency is temporarily suspended.

It is important not to frighten the child for, if it cries, inhalation may take place. If it is possible to see the object when the child opens its mouth, it should be grasped, either with the fingers or a pair of forceps or eyebrow tweezers, and gently removed. On no account should it be pushed further down the throat. An infant should be picked up by the heels and slapped on the back. If choking takes place, and there is spasm of the larynx, asphyxia may occur. In this emergency it may be necessary to carry out a *tracheostomy* (see p. 112). Once an adequate airway has been established, the acute emergency has ended and it is immaterial whether the child has voided the foreign body or not, since examination and investigation can be carried out later under the right circumstances with the right equipment. All vomited foreign bodies should be kept for inspection by the doctor.

Adults are less likely to inhale foreign bodies but may do so due to bad habits, such as holding safety pins and sewing pins between the lips whilst working. Foreign bodies which can cause trouble are fish bones, which being sharp can often embed themselves in the base of the tongue, tonsil and vallecular region but, if successfully passing these sites, can often end up in the pyriform fossae. Coins usually pass down into the oesophagus but may become stuck in the laryngeal region. Small dentures tend to stick in the oesophagus.

Intubation

This is an emergency measure carried out when asphyxiation is occurring. There may be an obstruction either above the larynx or in the larynx, or the asphyxiation may be caused by respiratory failure. It requires the minimum of preparation and apparatus and may be a life-saving measure. An endotracheal tube is introduced through the larynx and oxygen is supplied, either from a mechanical respirator or from the Boyle's anaesthetic apparatus, squeezing the bag rhythmically to stimulate normal respiration. The disadvantages of intubation are that it is only temporary and the tube may become blocked by dried secretions. Also, attempts at intubation may result in pushing the foreign body down into the lungs, resulting in inhalation infections.

Tracheostomy

This is a particularly useful measure if the obstruction is permanent or semipermanent, as in acute tracheo laryngitis of children and in acute bronchitis, and where the obstruction is in or near the glottic opening. It may be carried out under local or general anaesthetic, preferably in the operating theatre. An incision is made through the skin either in the mid-line or transversely, and the superficial fascia separating the pretracheal muscles is pulled to either side of the mid-line down to the trachea. There may be a small part of the thyroid gland joining the two lobes in front of the trachea and impeding the approach to its surface; this may be ligated or divided. A circular hole is made in the trachea anteriorly (Figure 77) below the first two rings from the cricoid. The tracheostomy tube is then inserted. An anaesthetic or respiratory apparatus can be connected to the tube to allow forced respiration to be carried out.

The tracheostomy tube may be made either of silver or plastic. A silver tube is an advantage when used with children, since its walls are thinner and it has an inner and outer tube. This allows a better flow of air than is obtained with a plastic tube, although the plastic tube is easier to look after and does not need changing so often. The tube should be the correct size for the patient. This is the surgeon's responsibility but the nurse should also check on it. The tube is attached by tapes passed round the patient's neck. They should be tight enough to keep it in place, but not so tight that they constrict the neck. They should be tied at the side of the patient's neck and the knot should be a double-bow knot which can be untied easily. The incision is usually sutured with silk or thin nylon, and surrounded with tulle gras impregnated with fucidin or penicillin. The

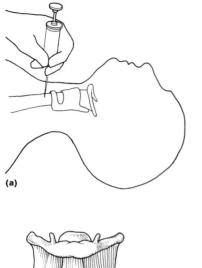

(a)

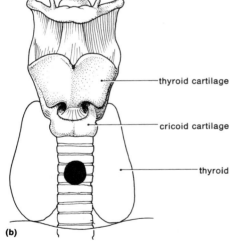

thyroid cartilage

cricoid cartilage

thyroid

(b)

Figure 77 Tracheostomy, showing (*a*) injection of local anaesthetic and (*b*) location of opening

skin of the neck and chest is protected from sputum, blood and secretions with a square of silk with a hole in it, and a little barrier cream is massaged into the neck and chest to help protect this region. A layer of one thickness of gauze should be laid over the orifice of the tube.

Nursing care

Particularly with children, there should always be a nurse on duty to care for the tracheostomy. She should have a sucker available with a catheter attached for removing secretions, and swabs and forceps. There should also be a spare plastic tracheostomy tube or an inner tube to fit the silver tube if this is being used. When the tube has to be changed, it should be replaced immediately with a new one, since, particularly in children, the wound tends to contract very rapidly. Feeding should be carried out with a feeding cup using small quantities at a time, since swallowing may be interfered with in the early stages. The surgeon decides the length of time the tracheostomy tube may be left in.

Acute oropharyngeal infections

These may be viral, bacterial or fungal in origin and may involve the whole of the oropharynx and spread up into the nasopharynx and down into the laryngopharynx and trachea. The most commonly seen infection of this nature is *tonsillitis*. In the acute phase, the tonsils become swollen and reddened, and yellow or whitish mucopus and sometimes a few specks of blood can be seen oozing from the crypts. There are certain special types of tonsillar infection. Thrush has already been mentioned (see p. 103). In *glandular fever*, a membranous film and rather cheesey debris is excreted from the crypts associated with brownish-red tonsils. This infection does not respond to antibiotics and is associated with enlarged lymph glands in the anterior and posterior triangles of the neck. The classical membranous tonsil infection, *diptheria*, is seldom seen in Great Britain today, thanks to widespread inoculation. In diphtheria, food and fluids may be regurgitated down the nose due to palatal paralysis interfering with digestion.

Occasionally, glandular fever may also produce this symptom, so diagnosis depends on pathological tests. Tuberculosis and syphilis, and certain of the granulomas, can also affect the oropharynx.

If the infection in the tonsils spreads through the capsule of the tonsil into the surrounding tissue, a condition called *peritonsillar abscess* or *quinsy* can arise (Figure 78). This is more common in adults where recurrent infections have led to the degeneration of the capsule of the tonsil. This unpleasant disease is painful and results in gross obstruction of the oropharynx. Sometimes the nasopharynx is completely blocked as well, causing upper respiratory obstruction. Treatment of this condition has been largely revolutionized by antibiotics but it is occasionally still necessary to open a quinsy (see p. 119).

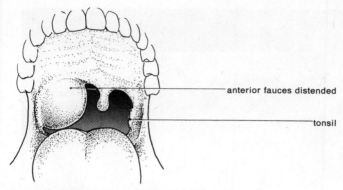

anterior fauces distended

tonsil

Figure 78 Peritonsillar abscesses or quinsy

Adenoidectomy and tonsillectomy

These are said to be the most frequently performed operations in modern surgery. Many different techniques may be used, usually depending on the surgeon. The sister in charge of the theatre is usually aware of the surgeon's preferred method.

The operations are usually carried out under general anaesthetic, given either with a Boyle–Davis gag attached to the anaesthetic apparatus so that the anaesthetic gases are delivered into the pharynx by a tube in the tongue plate, or through an endotracheal tube passed through the mouth. The adenoids atrophy with adolescence, so in adults, or younger patients whose adenoids do not need removal, the tube may be passed through the nose down into the trachea.

The adenoids are removed by a *curette* (Figure 79). This is an instrument with a sharp blade lying between the two wings of a curved wishbone. The blade is at right angles to the instrument and a backhanded sweep can remove the adenoids (Figure 80).

The tonsils are dissected from their bed, and sometimes ligatures are placed on bleeding points in the tonsillar fossae. These are usually of black silk and are left to slough away later. If haemorrhage is severe and difficult to control, the anterior and posterior pillars of the fauces may be sutured together with catgut (0 or 00). Very occasionally, it may be necessary to ligate the external carotid artery on the side of a bleeding tonsil.

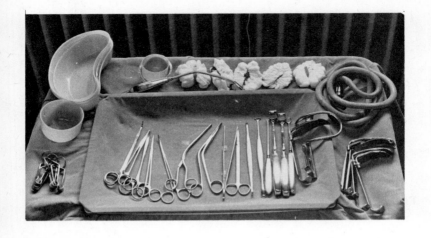

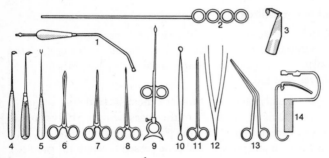

Figure 79 Instruments used for tonsillectomy.
1 Yankauer's tonsil suction tube; 2 Draffin suspension apparatus (one of two bipods); 3 Doughty's slotted endotracheal tongue plate; 4 St Clair Thomson adenoid curettes (guarded and unguarded); 5 Negus knot tier and ligature adjuster; 6 Negus tonsil artery forceps; 7 Birkett's fine tonsil artery forceps (curved); 8 Birkett's fine tonsil artery forceps (straight); 9 Eve's tonsil snare; 10 Mollison's semisharp enucleator; 11 Wilson's tapered and round-ended scissors; 12 Waugh's tenaculum dissection forceps; 13 Denis Brown's tonsil-holding forceps; 14 Davis gag and Boyle's tongue plate

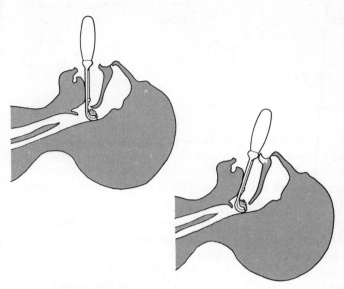

Figure 80 Adenoidectomy

Haemorrhage from the raw bed of the adenoids is relatively uncommon, but occasionally a swab must be placed in the post-nasal space to stop it. The technique is to pass a silk thread from the back of the nose to the anterior nose to hold the swab in place, and another may be led out through the mouth. The pack is removed after about 48 hours by this latter thread.

It is important to count the swabs before and after the operation, just as carefully as after an abdominal operation. If there is any discrepancy, the patient should not leave the operating theatre until the swab is found.

Nursing care
Post-operatively, the critical period lasts from the moment the patient leaves the operating theatre until he is fully conscious in the ward. The patient usually recovers consciousness fairly quickly, but he should not be allowed to leave the recovery room until he is conscious. During this time

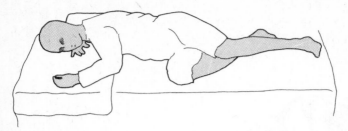

Figure 81 The post-anaesthetic (tonsillectomy) position

he should be continuously attended and kept lying on his right side until fully conscious, to prevent inhalation of blood and secretions (Figure 81). The major danger after any throat or nose operation is haemorrhage, with the possible consequence of inhalation of blood clot and debris, resulting in respiratory obstruction and suffocation.

After the operation, the patient should be observed for undue loss of blood from the nostrils, any tendency to swallow frequently associated with difficulty in breathing, change of colour or pulse, and vomiting of clots of blood. A suction apparatus, which should be pre-tested for efficiency, should always be available with a rubber-ended nozzle and catheter. However, the patient should not be interfered with too much, in case clots of blood are dislodged from the fossae and post-nasal space, which otherwise might help to produce haemostasis. A mouth gag, wooden jaw lever and a pair of sponge forceps with a swab on each should also be available for instant use. The airway left in by the anaesthetist should be kept in the mouth until the patient coughs it out himself. If undue oozing occurs, the surgeon may prescribe one of the coagulating drugs, such as *dicynene* to be administered intramuscularly. The instructions of the anaesthetist should be understood completely, and followed to the letter. A note should also be made of any post-operative drugs to be given. Help in emergency must be readily available during this part of recovery, for a few seconds can make all the difference between life and death.

Later signs of haemorrhage are rising pulse rate (although this will tend to rise anyway as the result of blood loss at operation and atropine as premedication), restlessness, obvious respiratory obstruction, swallowing and vomiting of blood. The time of the bleeding can also be estimated from the colour and consistency of the vomit; bright red blood means recent bleeding, dark clots indicate less recent haemorrhage. Vomited blood should always be kept and measured to help the surgeon in charge. The nurse should never be afraid to call for help if she is at all unhappy about the condition of the patient.

Quinsy

The swelling of quinsy may become so great that, if the condition involves both sides, respiratory obstruction can take place, associated with difficulty in swallowing and opening the mouth. The main treatment is to administer heavy doses of antibiotics. If possible, the infective organism should be cultured for sensitivity and the appropriate drug then used. Eventually, however, the abscess may come to a head, usually in the region of the anterior fauces. It may burst spontaneously, or it may require incision and drainage.

This is best carried out under local anaesthetic, for example, 10 per cent cocaine sprayed on to the pharynx. The patient is instructed to take several deep breaths and then hold his breath with the mouth wide open. The surgeon, wearing a head lamp, then makes an incision along the line of the fauces, with a guarded scalpel if necessary, afterwards dilating the incision with sinus forceps. The patient then spits out the blood, pus and debris into a large bowl (a towel should be covering the bed in case of accidental spills). A glass of mouthwash should be available. The condition then usually subsides with little trouble. Cultures should be made from the pus obtained, and the appropriate antibiotics then administered.

Laryngeal affections

Although infections of the larynx are described separately from those of the mouth, the whole of the pharynx is interconnected, and affections of one part will often involve another.

Simple *laryngitis* may be acute or chronic and is often secondary to an upper-respiratory infection. The larynx appears reddened and, because of some oedema of the vocal cords and surrounding structures, the voice becomes hoarse or absent and swallowing may be painful. Inhalations, if carried out at frequent intervals, may bring considerable relief (see p. 87). If the doctor has prescribed a regime of silence, the nurse should see that the patient obeys this and that he has writing materials so that he can communicate with those around him. Any other treatment prescribed by the doctor should be carried out regularly.

Acute laryngo-tracheo bronchitis

This condition may occur in epidemic form and can be particularly serious, since the whole of the respiratory tract is involved in a sudden acute infection which produces a particularly tenacious exudate. This exudate tends to form crusts made up of the desquamated epithelium of the respiratory passages, together with the exudate produced by the infection. Infants and young children in the toxic and pyrexial (feverish) condition which results from the severe infection are not strong enough to cough away these crusts, and the lungs can collapse, with associated laryngeal obstruction due to swelling of the tissues and blockage by secretions. This produces cyanosis and circulatory failure and may result in death. Tracheal intubation, tracheostomy (see p. 112) and bronchoscopy may be life-saving procedures in these cases.

Bronchoscopy is an important operation requiring the same care over sterilization etc. as any other theatre operation. Before the operation, the instruments should be tested and sterilized. The connecting flex, bulbs and bulb holders should be carefully checked. This requires especial care when using the older instruments involving the very tiny bulbs, usually about the size of a grain of rice. These are very delicate and must be tested gently and carefully, allowing the test current to build up slowly so that they do not blow. A more recent method of illumination consists of a high-intensity bulb working off the mains in a container with a lens system, leading to a flexible fibreglass head which carries the light to the end of the instrument. Different sizes of instrument should be prepared, sterilized and lubricated with liquid paraffin at the tip. Suitable suction tubes and swab holders should also be at hand. The swabs, which are very small, should be carefully counted before and after the operation.

Nursing care
Nursing care in these cases is extremely important. The child is sometimes in an oxygen tent, and the proper flow of oxygen must be maintained. There is a risk of asphyxia if the airway is not kept clear of secretions, and the breathing, pulse rate and colour of the child should be frequently noted, since anoxia (lack of oxygen) can rapidly cause intracranial damage. The nurse must make sure that a spare cylinder of oxygen is readily available.

If a tracheostomy has been carried out, the nurse must make certain that the tube is free of crusts and secretions at all times, and she should swab out any excess secretions which may be present. The natural functions of the bowels and bladder must also be cared for in the infant so that it spends the minimum time without oxygen.

Laryngeal obstruction and paralysis

The larynx may become obstructed by foreign bodies, but there are several other conditions which can cause laryngeal obstruction. It can be affected by local and external disease and also damaged by direct trauma, resulting from blows on the thyroid cartilage. This can cause collapse and severe oedema and bruising. Unarmed combat, attempted strangulation and road traffic accidents are all responsible for laryngeal injury.

The vocal cords may be paralysed on one side or bilaterally as a result of interference with the recurrent laryngeal nerves which supply the intrinsic muscles of the larynx. Should only one side be paralysed, complete obstruction will not occur and, even if both nerves are completely destroyed or non-functional, complete obstruction will not occur if the vocal cords are not oedematous. If there is no nerve supply at all to the larynx, the vocal cords remain in what is called the *cadaveric position*, where a narrow chink remains through which respiration can take place.

Among the diseases of the nervous system which cause laryngeal paralysis are bulbar palsy, acute polyneuritis and anterior poliomyelitis. Diseases of the chest can cause paralysis of the recurrent laryngeal nerves. Among the most important of these diseases are carcinoma of the lung and tuberculosis of the apical region. Fibrous tissue or malignant spread may involve the lower part of the nerve, first producing a mid-line paralysis of the cord and later, as the nerve becomes further involved, allowing the vocal cord to come to rest in the cadaveric position. The vocal cord on one side adjusts itself to the paralysis of the other.

The recurrent laryngeal nerve can also be damaged or destroyed during the operation of thyroidectomy. The inferior thyroid artery lies in close proximity to the nerve, which may be either crushed or severed during ligation of the blood vessel or removal of the gland. Paralysis of the vocal cord gives a hoarse voice, but does not obstruct respiration.

Laryngofissure

In this operation, one of the vocal cords is removed, together with the cartilage on the affected side. The patient is given a temporary tracheostomy but is eventually allowed to breath through the natural channels of the larynx if good healing takes place.

Laryngectomy

This operation consists of the removal of the whole larynx and some of the surrounding muscles. It is usually accompanied by a block dissection of the lymph glands in the neck. The pharynx is reconstructed by plastic surgery, enabling the patient to swallow food again. Operations involving removal of the larynx always result in a permanent tracheostomy, which requires careful attention in the post-operative period.

The surgeon in charge is responsible for the care of the patient during the first few days after the operation, and there must always be a special nurse in attendance. If the nurse has to leave the room, even for a short time, she should arrange for a replacement, since the patient cannot call for help if it is needed.

In the operation, the suture lines are complex and may be under some tension and there will usually be two drainage tubes.

The tracheostomy must be kept clean, and tracheal and bronchial infection prevented if possible by scrupulous attention to detail, aseptic precautions and antibiotic treatment. A tulle gras dressing is usually wrapped round the outer tracheostomy tube in a conical shape. A dressing trolley will be necessary with instruments, angular dressing, forceps, swab holders, swabs and dressing, and a sucker with a catheter ready for instant use. A cannula with an inner and outer tube is generally used post-operatively. An inner tube should always be kept ready sterilized. The patient is best nursed in an almost-sitting-up position. The inner tube should be removed every one or two hours, a replacement inserted, and the dirty tube cleaned, sterilized and placed on the bedside trolley for ready use.

When the stitches are healed, and the wound dry, a different tube of either metal or plastic may be used. Later, when the opening into the trachea (the *stomar*) is quite stable, and not liable to contract, the tube may be discarded. Some patients like to keep a tube in place for fear of the opening narrowing and closing.

Nursing care
Post-operative feeding is best carried out through an *oesophageal tube* through the nose. It is important to see that the patient does not pull this tube out when coming round from the anaesthetic. For the first 24 hours, nothing but water should be given, five or six times a day in quantities from 25 to 50 ml. Then, if all is well, the feed can be graduated to milk, Complan, and beaten-up egg with a little brandy and vitamins. The feeds

should be given before the dressings are changed, thereby showing any leakage present. This also means that the patient waits for the shortest possible time with wet uncomfortable dressings. The most common time for the wound to break down is about the twelfth day, when saliva or mucus leaking from the wound or drainage holes is a common sign. If there is a tendency to leakage, the dressings should be kept firmly in place with a fairly tight webbing and changed frequently. From the tenth to the fourteenth day, the patient may be allowed to swallow without the tube if no leakage is present.

Functional aphonia

This is a condition where the patient loses the ability to phonate, either due to psychogenic or hysterical causes. It can be distinguished from an organic hoarseness of the voice by the fact that, when asked to cough, the patient can cough quite normally, although normal speech appears impossible. Using the laryngeal mirror, the cords can be seen to be capable of normal approximation when coughing, but, during phonation, they are disorganized and indeterminate in their movement (see p. 107).

Corrosive fluids

The effects of the ingestion of corrosive fluids and poisons may be manifest throughout the whole of the upper respiratory and gastrointestinal tracts. Damage may occur anywhere from the lips to the oesophagus, but certain of the structures involved are more liable to damage than others.

Poisons may be swallowed accidentally by children and also by adults; although in adults there is always the additional possibility of a suicide attempt. The poison is liable to produce burns around the lips and the base of the tongue in the region of the valleculae and also in the pyriform fossae and larynx. These are places where fluid tends to pause during normal deglutition (swallowing) and, if the poison passes through the oesophagus, further burning can occur. Burning from corrosives may result in ulceration in all sites of the oesophagus and stenosis may occur in the normal narrowing parts at the oropharyngeal sphincter, behind the left bronchus and just above the cardiac orifice. The corrosive fluid may be delayed here, and therefore cause more damage.

The nurse, presented with a patient who has swallowed a poison or corrosive fluid, should try to identify the fluid ingested, and keep any bottle, vomit or cups, etc., which can be obtained. This will help to identify the substance and is also important from the medico-legal point of view.

The important measure is to neutralize the poison used. Acids should be treated with alkali, and vice versa, and the nurse should become familiar with the antidotes to common corrosive poisons.

Nursing care

The general care of pre-operative cases will not be discussed here but it is important to mention certain special aspects of ENT nursing which do not come into other fields.

The choice of parenteral pre-operative medication rests with the anaesthetist and his instructions should not only be precisely obtained and understood, but must be followed out to the letter at the exact time and in the exact quantities prescribed.

When premedicating children on an ENT list, a part of the premedication may sometimes be administered by mouth, and careful supervision should ensure that the children have really taken the drugs prescribed and not vomited or otherwise disposed of them. All drugs must be checked and signed for.

Summary of nursing points

The common infections of the pharynx, larynx and trachea include inflammatory conditions, such as tonsillitis, laryngitis and tracheitis, together with operations such as tonsillectomy, laryngectomy and tracheostomy.

The nurse should study the infections that are prone to occur in this area of the body, together with their potential serious consequences for the patient, which may include loss of voice, loss of speech, total obstruction and death from pneumonia. She should be adept at effecting prompt measures when faced with emergency situations, such as obstruction caused by foreign bodies, as in the inhalation of vomitus, or the swallowing of corrosive liquids.

She must never forget her role in supporting the patient, who may suffer from emotional stress following disease and dysfunction of these organs.

Chapter 8   The external ear

General structure of the ear

The external ears are structures which in man and most other animals are situated on either side of the head. This helps to locate the source of sounds. Loss of hearing in one ear can make this location very difficult in the same way that loss of an eye makes it difficult to judge the distance of an object.

Anatomically the external ear (Figure 82) consists of that part, projecting from the head, which acts as a collecting area for sounds, and the auditory canal which is a tube, made partly of cartilage and partly of bone, leading into the skull. At the end of this canal lies the eardrum or *tympanic membrane* (Figure 83), which is a thin structure made up of two layers of epithelium with blood vessels and supporting tissue lying between them.

Sound is made by intermittent compressions of the air. Depending on the frequency of the compressions, the sound alters. For example, the humming of a bee is a deeper sound than the high-pitched whine of a mosquito. Both sounds are produced by the wings of the insect beating the air and causing compressions, but the mosquito's wings beat the air much faster. A sound wave (a series of compressions) striking the tympanic membrane causes it to vibrate at exactly the same rate as the sound wave.

To the inside of the tympanic membrane is attached the *malleus*, which is the first of the chain of bony levers (*ossicles*) which transmit the sound across the middle ear, converting the compressions in the air to a mechanical movement. There are three bones in the chain, the malleus on the outside, next the *incus* and then the *stapes* (Figure 84). The ossicles are a set of levers designed to reduce the degree of movement produced on the tympanic membrane, and to increase the force of pressure exerted at the inner end of the chain. The innermost ossicle, the stapes (or stirrup) and its footplate, covers a structure in the medial wall of the middle ear called

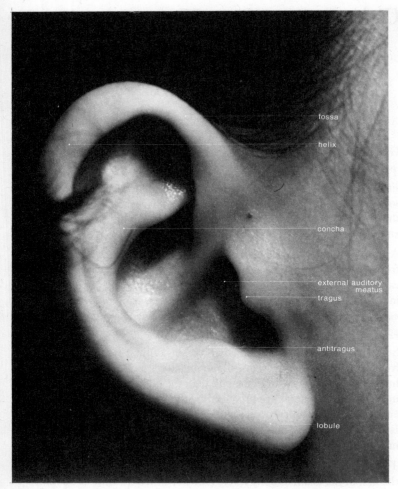

Figure 82 The external ear

the oval window or *foramen ovale*. Thus, a compression striking the tympanic membrane will be transmitted across the middle ear, via the malleus, incus and stapes, increased in force and reduced in amplitude to produce a movement inwards of the footplate of the stapes in the foramen ovale. The result of this is to produce a compression in the inner ear.

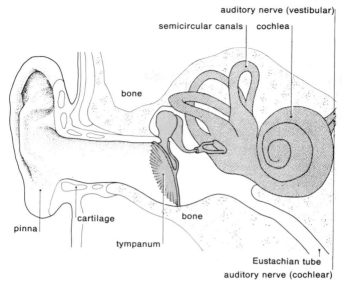

Figure 83 Section through the right ear

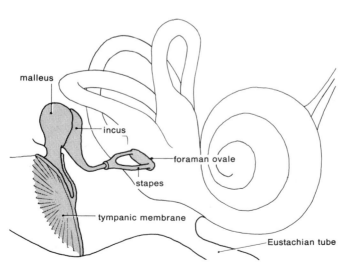

Figure 84 The tympanic cavity from the front

The inner ear contains fluid called *perilymph*. All fluid is incompressible, so the compression is transmitted throughout the perilymph system as a wave. The movement inwards of the foramen ovale is followed by a corresponding outward movement of another flexible membrane covering a round window lying anterior to the oval window, in the medial wall of the middle ear. The shock wave in the perilymph system stimulates the nerve endings in a special organ of hearing called the *organ of Corti*, which is surrounded by endolymph, and the nervous impulses are transmitted to the brain via the auditory nerve.

An important structure in the anterior and lower part of the middle ear is the *Eustachian tube* (see Figure 83). This leads from the middle ear to the nasopharynx and its purpose is to maintain the air pressure in the middle ear at the same level as that of the outside atmosphere. This is very important for, should the internal pressure be greater than that of the outside atmosphere, the membrane will bulge and lose its free movement. This will interfere with hearing and induce pain. If the pressure in the middle ear is less than the outside atmosphere, the tympanic membrane will be retracted, with similar interference with hearing and also pain.

Affections of the ear

The external ear can be afflicted with congenital abnormalities which may range from complete absence of the external ear to absent lobes and the deformity of *bat ears*. The middle ear may also suffer maldevelopments and the ossicular chain may be deformed or absent.

Trauma to the external ear is very common, and one of the best-known conditions is that of *cauliflower* ear. This results from *haematoma* (bruising), which may also become infected, occurring under the perichondrium of the cartilage which gives shape to the external ear. This skin is very close to the cartilage, and the tension produced in the haematoma is so great that the blood supply to the cartilage is interfered with, and the cartilage eventually atrophies, producing the characteristic deformity.

Foreign bodies of all sorts can be forced into the external canal and should be removed with great care, using the proper equipment, since damage can easily be done to the delicate structures of the tympanic membrane.

Blast injuries may damage the tympanic membrane, often splitting it down the line of the handle of the malleus. A blast injury may also injure the cochlea, by the passage of an excessive shock wave in the endolymph

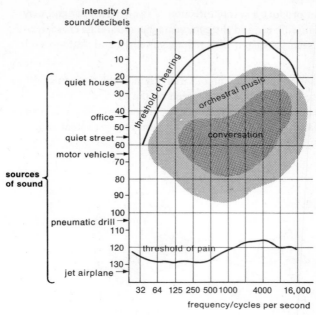

Figure 85 The limits of human hearing

crushing the organs of corti. This is particularly likely with sounds in the region of 4300 cycles (Figure 85) which strike the cochlea at the bottom of its spiral.

Fractures of the base of the skull may cause deafness through injury to the middle ear, or bleeding into it. Fractures which involve the temporal bone, by damaging the nerve supply to the labyrinth (see p. 134), may destroy both balance and hearing. Damage to the auditory nerve may also occur.

Infection of the external ear

This is very common. In addition, irritation in allergic states and anxiety may cause inflammation of the skin of the ears and post-auricular regions. The *aural furuncle* is often bacterial and staphylococcal in origin, and is an infection of a hair follicle in the external auditory canal. It is very painful and produces swelling in the canal and surrounding ear tissues, together with extreme tenderness of the external ear.

Herpes zoster can produce a severe infection of the external ear and may also involve the middle ear and the geniculate ganglion. The characteristic vesicles may be seen associated with redness, swelling and deafness and vertigo.

Virus myringitis is an inflammation of virus origin of the tympanic membrane where bulging areas can be seen on the surface of the membrane. Infections with *Bacillus proteus*, pyocyaneous and fungi can all be responsible for external ear infections, and are very persistent and difficult to treat.

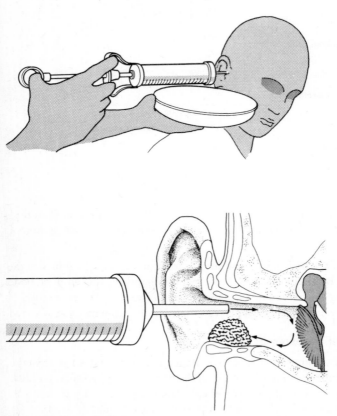

Figure 86 Ear syringing

Ear syringing

This is a minor procedure frequently carried out in an out-patient's department, although it needs great care and properly maintained equipment. The ear syringe is a 50 or 100 ml syringe with a nozzle which screws on to the end. This nozzle must be properly screwed home before use (Figure 86) since, if it comes off during syringing, it may be propelled into the external auditory meatus, causing damage not only to the meatus, but also possibly to the tympanic membrane, or even the inner ear by cracking the wall of the lateral semicircular canal. This may cause severe and possibly permanent deafness and vertigo. Infection may be introduced if the apparatus is not properly sterilized, and excessive force or clumsiness may result in pain and suffering. There is also an ear syringe which uses a right-angled nozzle attached to a Higginson's syringe. This has the advantage of being safer to use, but it is important to make sure that the bulb of the syringe is completely filled each time before compressing it, otherwise bubbles of air can be expressed through the nozzle. This produces a noise which the patient finds most unpleasant.

Summary of nursing points

The nurse should appreciate the role of the ear and its importance to the patient and realize that loss of hearing, either partial or complete, can produce marked emotional stress in the patient. Her supportive role in this situation is vital.

She should understand the common conditions which affect the external ear, i.e. congenital abnormalities, foreign bodies in the external auditory canal, *Herpes zoster* and furuncle. The nurse must become proficient in the procedure of syringing the ear, together with the instillation of medicament, should this be prescribed.

Chapter 9

The middle and inner ear

The inner ear

This is the part of the ear concerned with changing the physical movement of sound compressions into nervous impulses. It has two functions, hearing and balance. The organs of hearing and balance are both surrounded by perilymph fluid which flows between all the structures, but the two systems, the *cochlear* (hearing) and *vestibular* (balance) systems, have separate nervous connections. Both systems are affected in conditions where infection or malfunction of the perilymph flow takes place.

The cochlear and vestibular systems

These consist of an outer bony labyrinth filled with *perilymph* which surrounds an inner membranous labyrinth filled with *endolymph* (Figure 87). The sense organs are situated in this membranous labyrinth, in direct contact with the endolymph. Movement of the endolymph stimulates the end organs of the cochlear and vestibular branches of the eighth auditory nerve (see Figure 83), sending nervous impulses to the higher centres of the brain, the parts concerned with hearing and balance.

The *cochlea* is a spiral structure divided into three compartments. When compression occurs in the first compartment (in the perilymph) as a result of inward movement of the oval window, the shock waves cause the fluid in the cochlea to vibrate. The vibration is possible because the perilymph in the second compartment is continuous with the round window which bulges out when the foramen ovale is pushed in. The third compartment contains endolymph, and has sensitive receptors in the organ of corti. These react to stimulation by producing nervous impulses, which pass up the cochlear division of the eighth nerve to the brain.

It is thought that the apex of the cochlea is concerned with the lower-pitched sounds and that the lower turns of the cochlea are concerned with higher-pitched sounds.

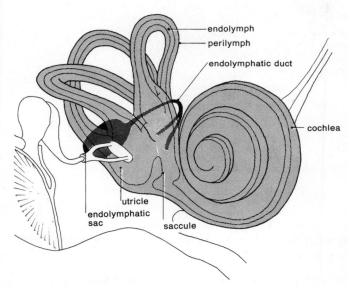

Figure 87 The endolymphatic system of the inner ear

The balancing mechanism

The balancing mechanism is rather more complex. The brain obtains its information about the position of the head in three main ways:

1 Lateral positional information is supplied from the maculae of the *saccule*;
2 Fore-and-aft positional information is supplied from the maculae of the *utricle*;

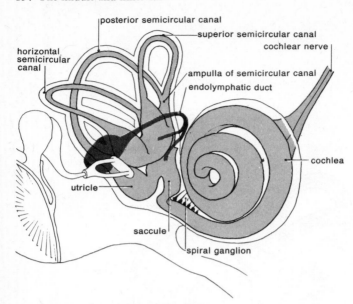

Figure 88 The membranous labyrinth

3 Rotational information is supplied by the three semicircular canals from the *ampullae* of each canal.

The maculae of the saccule and utricle are dilatations in these organs containing chalky particles in a collection of mucus. When the head is tilted to one side, the weight of the mucus and chalky particles pulls on the epithelium of the macula and stimulates the sensitive nerve endings contained in the epithelium. Nervous impulses are sent up the vestibular nerve and the information is interpreted by the vestibular nucleus and the rest of the brain.

For example, if the head is tilted to the right, the maculae of the right saccule will send out impulses; if the head is tilted forward, the maculae of the utricles will be stimulated together and send a message to the brain to say that the head is tilting forward.

There are three semicircular canals at right angles to each other, the *horizontal* (lateral), *superior* and *posterior* (Figure 88). At the start of each canal is the *ampulla* which corresponds to the maculae in the saccule or utricle. It contains the sense organs and nerve endings of the other part of the vestibular nerve. In this case, the sense organ is designed to react to fluid movements in the canals, rather like weed in a tidal river which points one way when the river is flowing down, and the other way when the tide is coming in. As the head rotates, the endolymph in the canal in the line of rotation lags behind the body and momentarily stimulates the end organs in the ampulla of that canal. The amount of stimulation is directly proportional to the acceleration of the head movement, and the corresponding canal in the other ear in the same plane will have a minimal response. These nervous impulses are all relayed to the vestibular nuclei and analysed by the brain. The whole complex system of the labyrinth is therefore linked to postural and stretch reflexes from other parts of the body and particularly from the eyes, enabling the individual to remain upright in the dark and on uneven surfaces.

Sea sickness is partly induced by confusion arising in the brain from a vast number of conflicting messages received from the eyes, legs, body and labyrinth together which completely deranges the communications system and overloads the brain, which goes into revolt and induces vomiting.

Injuries to the cervical spine

The *vertebral arteries*, paired blood vessels which contribute to the blood supply of the inner ear, run up through a canal in the cervical vertebrae from the fifth cervical vertebra upwards on both sides. They form the basilar artery which connects with the circle of Willis, from which is given off the *internal auditory artery*. Injuries to the cervical spine, and subsequent damage to the canals through which the blood vessels pass, may interfere with the blood supply of the labyrinths and produce vertigo and deafness.

Acute middle ear infection

The tympanic membrane can be perforated by foreign bodies which are forced into it from the outside, or by inflammation originating outside the membrane. However, perforation of the membrane most frequently results from infection inside the middle ear. The course of events consists firstly of the outpouring of serous fluid containing bacteria and white blood cells and pus cells. This fills up the middle ear, and the pressure there rises. Some of this infected mucopus and pus is then forced under pressure into the mastoid cells. Pressure on the tympanic membrane eventually causes bulging, and the blood vessels which lie between the two

Figure 89 Types of perforation of the tympanic membrane in chronic otitis media

layers of the membrane become occluded, resulting in necrosis or death of the area under pressure. This area then splits open, spilling the contents of the middle ear into the meatus, causing a discharge. The moment this occurs, the acute pain from the earache is instantly over. The infection may then subside completely, the tympanic membrane healing and hearing being restored to normal. However, in certain cases the middle ear remains infected, with drainage through a chronic perforation (Figure 89). This condition is known as *chronic supparative otitis media* and may continue for years. Sometimes operative procedure may be necessary to remove infection, produce a dry ear and preserve hearing.

If the tympanic membrane is particularly tough, the mastoid cells may become filled with infected mucopus. The infection can be controlled with antibiotics, and may subside, or it may drain through an adequate perforation in the tympanic membrane. Otherwise, the condition of mastoiditis may occur. An important factor here is whether the passage between the middle ear and the mastoid remains patent or not. If it becomes blocked by mucosal swelling or infected debris, there is only one course which the infection can take, and that is to break through the weakest of the boundaries surrounding it. This may be upwards into the brain, backwards into the lateral sinus or outwards into the subcutaneous tissues overlying the mastoid. In each case an abscess cavity may be formed which will have to be opened and drained. This is carried out by performing a *cortical mastoidectomy* operation.

Cortical mastoidectomy operation

In this procedure, an incision is made approximately one centimetre behind the junction of the posterior border of the ear with the scalp; this incision is carried down from the level of the external ear almost to the tip of the mastoid process. It is made deep enough to incise the periosteum covering the mastoid part of the temporal bone, and the skin and muscle flap is reflected backwards and forwards with a *rougine* (a form of chisel), exposing the bone itself. The periosteum is separated up to the margin of the bony meatus, but avoiding separation of the posterior wall of the meatus, since, if this occurs, a narrowing of the meatus may result after the operation.

The thin layer of bone covering the mastoid cells is then chipped away with a mallet, aiming at all times towards the position of the additus of the mastoid antrum. Great care is taken to avoid damaging the facial nerve which, in its vertical part, lies deep to the additus, and eventually emerges from the stylomastoid foramen. The more delicate parts of the clearance of diseased bone etc. are carried out under the operating microscope by means of an electric dental drill.

In children, the facial nerve lies quite close to the surface at the tip of the mastoid, and can easily be damaged. When the mastoid cells are exposed, the diseased bone is removed either with a gouge, nibbling forceps or a dental burr. As the diseased bone is removed, the lateral sinus can be exposed posteriorly and any abscess in that region drained. The dura mater can also be explored, and any abscess in the extradural space drained. An abscess in this region may extend into the subdural space, which may also then be drained. Medially, an abscess may exist in the petrous part of the temporal bone, or the zygoma region anterior to the middle ear. When the infected and diseased structures have been exposed, any diseased bone removed, the cavity produced made smooth and all pockets of infection opened up, the postaural wound is irrigated with hydrogen peroxide solution (10 vols) to clean out debris etc. The upper part of the incision is then closed with sutures and a drain of corrugated rubber or plastic inserted into the inferior part of the wound. A mastoid head bandage is then tied to hold the dressings in place. This consists of a strip of tulle gras over the incision, the gauze and, lastly, a pad of cotton wool.

Dressings are left in place for 24 hours and then the top dressing is removed with the discharges etc. When the discharge subsides, the drainage tube may be partially or completely removed, *according to the surgeon's instructions*, and a dry dressing replaced. An antibiotic cover, either with penicillin or an appropriate antibiotic, is usually given for a week or ten days. The sutures, commonly silk or nylon, are removed on the seventh day, or alternate sutures may be left in for two or three days more. The wound should be healed in a fortnight and any discharge from the tympanic membrane should have ceased. The first post-operative dressing should be carried out by the surgeon, who will note any oedema or signs of infection. If there is discharge, swabs should be taken for sensitivities to allow the antibiotic cover to be changed. Successive dressings may be done by nursing staff, and usually consist of a gauze dressing with a cotton wool pad. The external auditory meatus may be swabbed with spirit and cotton wool, and the drainage tube shortened in one-centimetre lengths as dressings are carried out.

Radical mastoidectomy operation

This is an operation for chronic suppurative otitis media which becomes necessary when the chronic infection has advanced to such a stage that the contents of the middle ear are largely destroyed. In fact, the middle ear cavity may become occupied by *cholesteatoma* (a mass of debris made up of desquamated epithelium shed by the walls of the middle ear) which has become confined within the cavity. At times, as the condition progresses, steady erosion of the bony walls can take place, exposing and destroying the vital structures which surround the middle ear, such as the facial nerve, the lateral sinus, the dura mater and the labyrinth of the inner ear. This may result in facial paralysis, meningitis and acute vertigo. If infection should supervene in the presence of this debris (the cholesteatoma), a particularly foul-smelling discharge may occur, often due to anaerobic organisms (*B. proteus* and *pyocyaneus*) which can live comfortably in a confined space with no oxygen supply.

The operation has been considerably modified over the last twenty years. Originally it was designed primarily to produce a dry and safe ear following chronic infection, but in recent years attention has increasingly been paid to preserving the hearing as far as possible. Operations have been designed to reconstitute the tympanic membrane and, to some extent, the ossicular chain, by plastic inserts, thereby improving the conduction of sound across the middle ear. The contents of the attic of the middle ear are involved in chronic infection and these may often need to be cleaned out during operations on the chronic ear. This procedure does not necessarily interfere with hearing.

Nursing care

The post-operative care involves looking after the packs in the external auditory meatus and the dressings. The precise instructions should be given by the surgeon. However, in all cases, scrupulous care must be taken to avoid introducing infection into the operated area, and full aseptic precautions should always be taken when doing mastoid dressings.

Lateral sinus thrombosis

Severe infection in the mastoid may result in a thrombosis of the lateral sinus, a severe condition. In this case, the sinus must be opened and plugged to prevent spread of infection.

Serous otitis media

This condition, also known as secretory otitis media or 'glue ear', is the result of the treatment of recurrent nasopharyngeal infections with antibiotics. When treatment with antibiotics is carried out, the mucous membrane of the walls of the infected middle ear and Eustachian tube undergo a change in which the number of mucosal cells producing serous fluid increases. The middle ear and Eustachian tube become filled with a thick glutinous sterile fluid resembling condensed milk. This produces deafness of a middle ear type which, if untreated, may develop later into an adhesive otitis media causing permanent impairment of hearing.

The treatment of this condition is to incise the tympanic membrane under general anaesthetic and suck out the glutinous material. This improves the aeration of the middle ear. In certain cases a small plastic grummet may be inserted (using a microscope) into the anterior or posterior inferior quadrant of the tympanic membrane. This remains patent and preserves the necessary aeration of the middle ear. These grummets may be left in place until they are extruded into the external auditory meatus, after which the tympanic membrane heals. Alternatively, they may be removed, also using a microscope.

Nursing care

The main post-operative nursing treatment involves giving ear drops as directed by the surgeon, keeping cotton wool in the external auditory meatus if required, and removing the bandage covering the ear at the right time. When instilling drops into the ear, the patient should be lying on his side and the dropper is either inserted into the meatus or held several centimetres above it. About three drops should be instilled and the pinna then massaged to remove air from the meatus and to allow the drops to reach the inner part of the external auditory canal.

Otosclerosis

This is a condition of middle ear deafness which is believed to be of hereditary origin. It occurs more frequently in middle life and, in women, appears to be made worse by successive pregnancies. It is due to a growth of bone which covers and makes immobile the foramen ovale in the medial wall of the middle ear. This in turn immobilizes the stapes and interferes with the conduction of the sound waves across the middle ear. This condition results in a severe conductive deafness. As the condition progresses and the round window becomes involved, some degeneration of the cochlea may take place. This is because the immobility of the foramen ovale produces rises in pressure in the endolymph, and this damages the delicate structures of the organ of corti. The result of this is a progressive reduction in nerve perception.

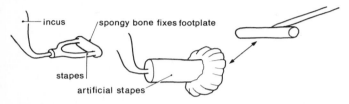

Figure 90 Stapedectomy, showing artificial stapes lying in the opening made in the stapes bone

Stapedectomy

The treatment of otosclerosis is by means of the operative procedure of *stapedectomy*. This operation has been developed continuously and consists of making a small window in the footplate of the stapes and inserting a specially made Teflon piston of a size designed to fit (Figure 90). This, in turn, is linked to the long process of the incus. The piston is surrounded by gel foam material.

The advantages of this operation are that the ear is unmarked, there is great improvement in hearing, minimal trauma occurs, the convalescence is short, and there is not a great deal of discomfort and vertigo after the operation. It is important that scrupulous aseptic care is observed. The incidence of sensori neural deafness following this operation is less than with some of the earlier techniques. Occasionally the piston may become displaced but it may be possible to re-open the ear and replace the prosthesis in position. Post-operative dressings are normally done by the house surgeon. The meatus is packed with 'calgetex' gauze or something similar.

After the operation, the patient should be warned that he may have some giddiness and that he should avoid blowing his nose too hard (he should only blow one side at a time). No water must get into the ear until healing has taken place. The patient should also avoid exposure to loud noises, because the stapedius muscle has been severed, thereby depriving the ossicular chain of its shock-absorbing effect, and allowing vibration to pass unchecked from the tympanic membrane to the inner ear. Football and boxing are unwise sports in which to indulge, but flying, tennis, golf and squash are quite permissible.

Other affections of the middle and inner ear
Neoplasms of the middle ear

Carcinoma can affect the middle ear, and treatment is by radical excision. The loss of function resulting from this surgery is a secondary consideration to the successful eradication of the neoplastic tissues.

Congenital conditions of the middle and inner ear

The structures of the middle ear may be affected in intra-uterine life, resulting in malformation of the ossicles and even complete absence of the middle ear structure. The inner ear may suffer malformation or complete maldevelopment.

Trauma to the middle ear and inner ear

This occurs particularly in fractures of the temporal bone. A microscopic fracture can result in an effusion of blood into the middle ear, and rupture of the tympanic membrane can take place, particularly when the bony part of the external auditory meatus is involved when the base of the skull is fractured. This can produce a blood-stained discharge from the middle ear and even cerebrospinal fluid can leak out into the external auditory meatus. Blast injuries can also produce direct damage to structures of the middle and inner ears.

Ménières syndrome

This is a condition of *vertigo* associated with vomiting and deafness, resulting from an intermittent malfunction of the endolymph system. It is thought to be due to a rise in pressure in the endolymph system, either due to excessive production of endolymph or to poor absorption. The original case was due to a haemorrhage into the labyrinth, but it is more likely that the syndrome is due to one or other of several conditions. Viral infections of the labyrinth and eighth cranial nerve can produce very similar clinical conditions, and encephalitis, which is a virus infection of the brain, can also produce vertigo.

When medical methods of treatment have failed, it may be necessary to destroy the labyrinth completely. When this has been done, the symptoms usually subside and the other labyrinth takes over. The operation is *labyrinthectomy*. An opening is made into the lateral semicircular canal and the membranous labyrinth is pulled out. An alternative procedure is to inject 100 per cent alcohol into the labyrinthine spaces, destroying the labyrinth. Sometimes the vestibular branch of the eighth cranial nerve is sectioned.

Labyrinthectomy is also carried out when labyrinthitis has been caused by infection spreading from the middle ear into the vestibular system. This may be linked with an otogenic brain abscess, which is an abscess which either occurs outside the brain lining, but inside the skull, or it may have spread into the substance of the brain. Infection may reach this region either via the middle ear or carried in the blood.

Neoplasms of the eighth nerve

The eighth nerve can be affected by the tumour, *acoustic neuroma*, and the symptoms vary depending on the part of the nerve involved. If the cochlear branch is involved, nerve deafness occurs and if the vestibular branch is involved then vertigo may be a principal symptom.

Von Recklinghausen's disease (or neurofibromatosis) is a condition where multiple nodular lesions occur on the nerves of the skin. Where a similar nodule occurs on the eighth cranial nerve, it can be a cause of eighth-nerve tumour.

Minor procedures

There are a number of minor procedures on the ear which may be carried out in the out-patient's department.

Catheterization of the Eustachian tubes

This is carried out to improve the aeration of the middle ear by blowing air through a tube called a *Eustachian catheter*. This is passed down the floor of the nose under local anaesthetic to the nasopharynx and inserted into the orifice of the Eustachian tube. The position of the tube in the orifice is checked by listening to the sound of air being blown through the tube by means of a stethoscope, placed with one end in the patient's external ear and the other in the surgeon's ear. At the moment when the catheter enters the Eustachian orifice, and air is blown into the ear from a rubber bulb attached to the catheter by a tube, the sound heard changes character, and the air can be heard rushing into the middle ear. It can even be felt if the tympanic membrane is perforated. The local anaesthetic used is 10 per cent cocaine HCl solution, first sprayed into the nose. After a few minutes, a swab soaked in 10 per cent cocaine is inserted into the nostril and passed gently back along the nose to the orifice of the Eustachian tube and left there for a few minutes.

Cautery of the ears

Sometimes in the treatment of chronically discharging ears or following mastoid operations, granulations may form in the depth of the meatus or middle ear and it is sometimes necessary to cauterize these granulations. A solution of silver nitrate (10 per cent or 50 per cent) or sometimes a fused bead of solid silver nitrate on the end of a silver probe may be used. Alternatively, a saturated solution of trichloracetic acid may be used. All caustic fluids should be in glass-topped bottles and the fused beads of caustic should be kept either in special containers or burned up in a spirit flame. Silver nitrate stains the fingers and nails brown, so care should be taken when cleaning the instruments used in cauterization of the external and middle ear.

Tests for labyrinthine function

A physiological test of the function of the labyrinth which has considerable importance in diagnosis of vestibular disease is the 'warm and cold water caloric test'. The test depends on the fact that, when the ear is syringed with water a temperature-change will be transmitted to the labyrinth of the semicircular canals. The lateral semicircular canal is inclined at an angle of 30° from the horizontal in a forward direction. If the patient's head is tilted back at an angle of 60° from the vertical, this canal will then become vertical. Since warmer fluid rises, when water above body temperature is syringed into the ear, the endolymph will move upwards in the canal and if the water is colder it will move downwards.

The test makes use of a phenomenon known as *nystagmus*. This is a reflex movement of the eye to keep moving objects in view. The reflex is partly under the control of the labyrinth of the ear. In the normal ear, on stimulation with hot water, the eye should be drawn slowly across towards the flow of endolymph and then released in a flickering motion (nystagmus) towards the other side. For example, if the left ear is stimulated with hot water, the eye will move slowly across to the right and then will flick quickly back to the left. With cold water, the opposite should happen. Thus with hot water, nystagmus takes place to the same side; with cold water nystagmus takes place to the opposite side.

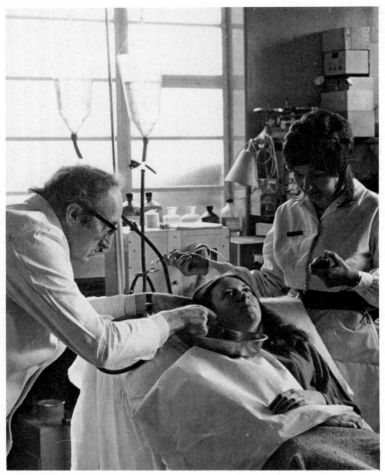

Figure 91 The caloric test

If the vestibular apparatus is dead or damaged, there may be no movement at all, or nystagmus of a much less marked degree. The water is used at two temperatures, one above and the other equally below the normal body temperature of 37 °C, i.e. at 44 °C (warm) and 30 °C (cold).

Reduced vestibular function may in itself produce a nystagmus to the opposite side from the lesion, whilst inflammation may produce a nystagmus to the same side.

Before caloric tests are performed, it is important that the ears are examined to ensure that both tympanic membranes are intact. If there is a perforation, caloric tests should not be carried out.

The patient is laid on an examination couch with his head at 30° from the horizontal (Figure 91). Water is kept in a thermostatically controlled bath about half a metre above the patient's head. The water inside is maintained at exactly 30 °C or 44 °C, and about two metres of rubber tubing lead from the bath with a nozzle on the end with a diameter such that not less than 200 g water will flow through in 40 seconds.

Some water is allowed to run through the nozzle into a bucket to bring the temperature of the outflowing water to that of the cold bath. Then the nozzle is inserted into the patient's ear and water is run in for exactly 40 seconds and the tube is clipped and removed. The patient is told to stare at a fixed point, and the time taken for the induced nystagmus to

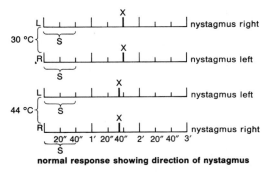

normal response showing direction of nystagmus

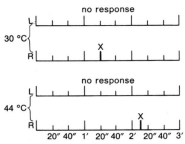

response in total loss of left vestibular function

Figure 92 The response to the caloric test.
The standard stimulation time (S) is 40 seconds

subside is measured with a stop watch. Five minutes elapse before the warm water test is started. The results are then plotted and assessed (Figure 92).

Other tests of labyrinthine function are the following:

1 *Cold air caloric tests.* These are used when there is damage to the middle ear, due to perforation, mastoid operation or some other operation on the middle ear cavity. A jet of cold air is blown into the ear. If no nystagmus is produced within 30–60 seconds, the labyrinth is considered to be inactive.

2 *Electronystagmography.* This is an electrical method of measuring nystagmus. Electrodes are placed near the outer canthus of the eye, and they measure changes in electrical potentials in the retina. The results are drawn on a graph using a recording galvanometer.

3 *Rotation in Bárány's chair.* This is another method of producing nystagmus. The patient is rotated rapidly for 20 seconds and then stopped. The duration of nystagmus produced indicates the degree of function of the labyrinth.

Hearing tests

These are carried out in the out-patient's department. Basically, the tests involve ascertaining the amount of hearing present and whether any hearing loss is due to abnormality of the middle ear (referred to as *conductive loss*), or *perceptive* loss, which is due to damage to the inner ear or auditory nerve. *Weber's test* consists of placing a tuning fork (512 Hz or 256 Hz) on the vertex of the skull.

1 If the hearing is normal, the patient will hear the sound in the centre of the head.

2 In middle ear (conductive) deafness, the patient will hear the sound more prominently in the *affected* ear.

3 In inner ear (perception) deafness, the sound will be heard more prominently in the *unaffected* ear.

Rinné's test is a further test which may be necessary. In this test, the tuning fork is place alternately just outside the external auditory meatus (to measure *air conduction*) and against the tip of the mastoid process (to measure *bone conduction*).

1 In normal hearing, air conduction is greater than bone conduction.

2 In middle ear deafness, bone conduction is greater than air conduction.

3 In inner ear deafness, air conduction may be equal to or greater than bone conduction.

The final test which can help distinguish middle ear deafness is the *absolute bone conduction test*. In this test, the tuning fork is placed against the patient's mastoid process with the meatus occluded. When the patient can hear the sound no longer, the tuning fork is immediately transferred to the tester's mastoid process, also with the meatus occluded. If the tester can hear the sound, this indicates that the patient has reduced nerve perception assuming that the examiner's hearing is normal.

Audiometry

This is a method of measuring a patient's loss of hearing in a more accurate way than can be done by clinical tests. There are several different types of audiometer. Some are automatically recording, and some assess the patient's hearing by producing a series of words at a given level of intensity (speech audiogram). The patient repeats the words that he recognizes and the correct results are recorded, as a percentage of the

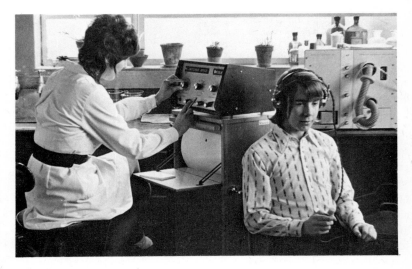

Figure 93 An audiometer

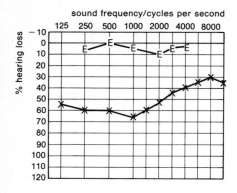

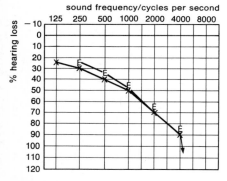

Figure 94 Audiograms.
Note that, in *conductive deafness*, there is a wide gap between nerve perception (E) and air conduction (X). In *perceptive deafness* nerve perception follows closely on the air conduction

total. The pure-tone audiometer is an electrical machine (Figure 93) which produces a series of pure sounds ranging in frequency from 125 cycles per second to 12 000 cycles per second. It has a device to reduce the intensity of the sound by five-decibel stages from 0 to 100. The intensity which allows a normal person to first hear the sound produced is considered as 0, and therefore the loss in hearing can be demonstrated in decibels. The tests are carried out in a quiet room and testing of both the air and bone conduction may be carried out, masking either ear by producing an irritating sound in the ear from the audiometer.

The nurse should understand the working of the audiometer in use, and make sure that there are no loose connections. She should ensure that the apparatus is ready for use, and if it runs off the mains, it must be connected and switched on as required. There should also be a form ready for use.

For the sake of uniformity, the convention has been adopted that, on the audiogram (Figure 94), for air conduction, the symbol 0 shall indicate the right-ear findings and X the left-ear findings. Various symbols are used to show nerve perception, for example:

Ǝ = right-nerve perception

E = left-nerve perception

or O and X in coloured pencil.

Masking is a technique which is used when air conduction and nerve perception in one ear is very low and in the other is normal. A continuous sound of variable strength is produced in the ear which is not being tested. This prevents transference of the sound from the audiometer through the bones of the skull which can lead to a false impression of hearing in the ear being tested.

The Impedence Meter

This is an instrument which measures the pressure inside the middle ear and from the readings produced, the presence of fluid in the middle ear, i.e. serous otitis and malfunctioning of the Eustachian tube, can be deduced. Certain other conditions e.g. fixation of the ossicles, otosclerosis, or undue flaccidity of the tympanic membrane, can also be ascertained. Nurses would not normally be expected to handle this instrument but they should at least know of its existence.

Summary of nursing points

The nurse should become proficient in the skills of observing the patient with suspected or actual disease of the middle and inner ear, such as mastoiditis, otitis media and otosclerosis. She should become conversant with the particular nursing care of the patient required to undergo surgery, i.e. mastoidectomy, labyrinthectomy and stapedectomy. She should become proficient in nursing procedures that may be indicated, such as instilling of medication, together with assisting the doctor in the preparation and carrying out of tests and examinations, such as cold air caloric tests. The nurse should understand the structure and functions of the middle and internal ear, and be aware of the close proximity of the inner ear to the brain; this is of particular importance in infections and during surgery of the middle and internal ear.

Further reading

General books

J. Darwin and J. Markham, *Eye, Nose, Throat and Ear Nursing: An Introduction*, Heinemann, 1966. A small book written to help nurses understand the more common conditions and procedures. The anatomy and physiology is investigated with the disorders in each part.

I. M. Duguid and A. A. Berry, *Ophthalmology*, EUP, 1971. A concise and explicit account of the diseases of the eye, each part preceded by its anatomy and each disease by its treatment. Nursing procedures and care complete the book, which also has a full glossary.

S. Duke-Elder, *Parsons's Diseases of the Eye*, 15th edn, Churchill, 1970. A comprehensive reference book.

E. H. M. Foxen, *Lecture Notes on Diseases of the Ear, Nose and Throat*, 3rd edn, Blackwell Scientific, 1972. Symptoms, signs and treatment of common conditions. Though written for doctors, this is clearly and simply written and is suitable for reference.

W. J. I. Fraser of Lonsdale, *My Story of St Dunstan's*, Harrap, 1961. A history of St Dunstan's. What can be done to overcome the handicap of blindness.

I. S. Hall and B. H. Colman, *Diseases of the Nose, Throat and Ear: A Handbook for Students and Practitioners*, 8th edn, Livingstone, 1967. Intended for doctors, but this is a good reference book for nurses. The anatomy of each part is followed by the disorders and treatment in clear, logical order. A chapter on endoscopy.

H. Ludman, *Ear, Nose and Throat Diseases: Principles of Patient Care*, Pitman, 1969. Diseases are described and the treatment of each, with emphasis on the understanding of the basic principles underlying it.

J. L. C. Martin-Doyle, *A Synopsis of Ophthalmology*, 4th edn, John Wright, 1971. A comprehensive view of ophthalmology in one small volume. For reference. Each part of the eye dealt with separately with anatomy and physiology, signs, symptoms and treatment.

Office of Health Economics, *The Ophthalmic Service*, Office of Health Economics, 1970. Development of the ophthalmic profession. Eye care under the Health Services. The provision of ophthalmic services and their cost.

P. Reading, *Common Diseases of the Ear, Nose and Throat*, 4th edn, Churchill, 1966. Written for doctors. This book provides a clear but comprehensive study of the ear, nose and throat and their disorders.

N. Roydhouse, *Ear, Nose and Throat Surgery for Students of Nursing*, Peryer, Christchurch, New Zealand, 1971. A simple account of the main diseases of the ear, nose and throat, the operations performed and the care required.

P. D. Trevor-Roper, *Lecture Notes on Ophthalmology*, 4th edn, Blackwell, 1971. A concise illustrated account of the common eye conditions and their treatment, though no actual nursing.

Chapter 1
Books

S. Duke-Elder, *Parsons's Diseases of the Eye*, 15th edn, Churchill, 1970. Chapters 1 to 9 give a detailed account of the anatomy and physiology of the eye, with some elementary optics, refraction, and methods of accommodation.

W. P. Gowland and J. Cairney, *Anatomy and Physiology for Nurses*, 7th edn, Peryer, Christchurch, New Zealand, 1965. Chapter 12 (pp. 212–30) outlines the anatomy and physiology of the eye – vision and accommodation.

G. L. McCullock, *Man Alive: A Survey of Human Physiology*, Aldus Books, 1967. Chapter 9 (pp. 98–106) describes the structure of the eye, with physiology of sight focusing and accommodation. Many excellent illustrations.

J. S. Ross, and K. J. W. Wilson, *Foundations of Anatomy and Physiology*, 3rd edn, Churchill Livingstone, 1968. Chapter 16 (pp. 410–20) discusses the anatomy and physiology of the eye, its muscles and accessory organs.

Chapter 2
Books

British Broadcasting Corporation, *In Touch: Aids and Services for Blind and Partially Sighted People*, BBC Publications, 1973. A practical guide to how to get help, money and employment, getting around, reading and working, everyday living and leisure, housing and holidays for the blind.

G. T. W. Cashell and I. M. Durran, *Handbook of Orthoptic Principles*, 2nd edn, Churchill Livingstone, 1971. Simple description of the principles involved in the management of squint.

P. Garland, *Ophthalmic Nursing*, 5th edn, Faber, 1960. Common eye investigations and treatments. Nursing of patients in casualty, out-patients and ward, with notes on work in the ophthalmic theatre.

L. Lurie, *Cataracts*, Foyle, 1962. A popular short account of types of cataract, how it affects people and operations for it and after-care.

World Health Organization Study Group, *The Prevention of Blindness*, Technical Report Series, no. 578 WHO Geneva, 1973. The extent of the problem of blindness – its causes and prevention etc.

Articles

J. D. Abrams, 'The nature of glaucoma', *Nursing Times*, vol. 68, 22 June 1972, pp. 767–70. A discussion of the causes, primary and secondary, and methods of treatment of this condition.

E. J. Arnott, 'Ultrasonic technique for removing the cataractous lens', *Nursing Mirror*, vol. 136, 2 Feb. 1973, pp. 27–8. An account of the technique – with its great advantage of short convalescence for the patient.

M. A. Bedford, 'Retinoblastoma', *Nursing Times*, vol. 68, 23 March 1972, pp. 340–43. An account of how, using modern methods of examination and treatment, this tumour may be eradicated.

R. L. Belsey, 'Do you think you need glasses? Or sight testing explained', *Nursing Times*, vol. 67, 21 Oct. 1971, pp. 1303–6. An account of what is entailed in sight testing and how results are interpreted.

A. Campbell, 'Tumours of the eye and orbit in childhood' (the second of a series of articles from the Royal Marsden Hospital), *Nursing Mirror*, vol. 134, 19 May 1972, pp. 26–9. Different types of tumours. Treatment aiming at saving sight as well as life.

D. P. Choyce, 'Intra-corneal plastic implants', *Nursing Times*, vol. 66, 4 June 1970, pp. 715–18. The plastic implant as an alternative to corneal grafting. Choice of implant, surgical routine and possible complications.

D. P. Choyce, 'Intraocular implants', *Nursing Times*, vol. 66, 28 May 1970, pp. 680–82. The use of perspex implants to replace lenses, preparation for operation – the operation described with after-care and possible complications.

L. H. Collier, 'Trachoma', *Nursing Times*, vol. 58, 6 April 1962, p. 428. An account of the history, nature and cause of the disease.

W. J. I. Fraser of Lonsdale, 'Psychological effects of blindness', *Rehabilitation*, April/June 1969, pp. 5–9. An account of the way in which these may be overcome. An understanding of the blind man's view of life.

W. Froëlich, 'That the sightless may see', *World Health*, Aug./Sept. 1972, pp. 12–17. An illustrated account of the different devices which help a blind person.

R. Gillon, 'Cataract – lifting the veil', *World Health*, June 1970, pp. 16–21. A clear account of the causes of cataract, symptoms, treatment and rehabilitation.

I. Jones-Ashton, 'Microscopes in ophthalmology', *Nursing Times*, vol. 68, 10 Feb. 1972, pp. 173–5. New fields opened up by use of microscopes in both treatment and teaching.

A. S. Kochar, 'India is tackling trachoma', *World Health*, June 1970, pp. 11–15. A picture story of the way India is trying to control trachoma.

R. J. McWilliam, 'Infection of the eye', *Nursing Times*, vol. 69, 1 Feb. 1973, pp. 145–6. The diagnosis and treatment of conjunctivitis, corneal abrasions and corneal ulcer.

S. Moday, 'Detachment of the retina. A cure is now possible', *World Health*, June 1970, pp. 28–33. A history of the understanding of this condition, predisposing factors, treatment and prevention.

P. Pereira, 'Screening for glaucoma', *Nursing Times*, vol. 68, 22 June 1972, pp. 771–4. The value of a trained ophthalmic nurse in the screening of patients so that unsuspected glaucoma may be recognized.

J. Reinhards, 'Flies, sand and trachoma', *World Health*, Jan. 1970, pp. 9–10. The attack on the cause and dissemination of trachoma.

M. Ruben, 'Contact lenses, shells and prosthetics', *Nuring Times*, vol. 68, 3 Feb. 1972, pp. 133–6. The use and value of these in many eye conditions. Some abnormalities resulting from wearing contact lenses.

M. Ruben, 'Contact lenses today', *Nursing Mirror*, vol. 125, 19 Jan. 1968, pp. 6–9. The use and value of contact lenses. The 'advice' on wearing them and the hygienic measures needed.

K. Rubinstein, 'Ophthalmic cryosurgery', *Nursing Times*, vol. 63, 8 Dec. 1967, pp. 1640–42. The use of extreme cold in surgical procedures, e.g. lens extraction, treatment of retinal detachment and glaucoma.

P. V. Rycroft, 'The modern management of retinal detachment', *Nursing Mirror*, vol. 123, 21 Oct. 1966, pp. 1–3. The purpose of treatment and the various techniques.

P. V. Rycroft, 'Modern trends of corneal grafting and its nursing problems', *Nursing Mirror*, vol. 126, 5 April 1968, pp. 19–22. Early attempts at corneal grafting with their nursing problems. Modern advances.

B. A. Samuel, 'Corneal grafting', *Nursing Times*, vol. 69, 1 March 1973, pp. 268–71. The value of this operation and the problems of obtaining donors.

P. J. H. Sellers, 'Glaucoma' (*Nursing Mirror* conference lecture), *Nursing Mirror*, vol. 131, 4 Sept. 1970, pp. 20–23. A description of the three main kinds of glaucoma and the lines of treatment adopted for each.

P. J. H. Sellers, 'Senile cataract', *Nursing Times*, vol. 64, 4 Oct. 1968, pp. 1337–9. Explanation of indications for operative treatment, the operation itself and the nursing care of the patient.

N. L. Simpson, 'Acrylic implants: a new vision', *Nursing Times*, vol. 126, 9 Feb. 1968, pp. 170–71. An account of the treatment of congenital cataract by an acrylic implant and of the subsequent restoration not only of sight but also of confidence in the patient.

A. Sorsby, 'Blindness in childhood', *Nursing Times*, vol. 64, 5 July 1965, pp. 903–4. An account of the causes of blindness in childhood. Comparison between causes during the last seventy years.

P. D. Trevor-Roper, 'Cataracts', *British Medical Journal*, vol. 3, 4 July 1970, pp. 33–5. Presenting features – medical treatment, indications for surgical treatment and methods of cataract removal and restoration of sight.

K. P. Whitehead, 'Chemical burns of the eye', *Nursing Times*, vol. 67, 24 June 1971, pp. 759–62. Incidence, prevention and treatment of these injuries.

Film

A film on corneal grafting may be obtained from the Corneoplastic Unit, Queen Victoria Hospital, East Grinstead.

Chapter 3
Books

A. S. Grimble, *McLachlan's Handbook of Diagnosis and Treatment of Venereal Diseases*, 5th edn, Livingstone, 1969. Page 22 gives a brief list describing affectation of the eye in late syphilis, while p. 89 briefly describes (with photographs of patients) the eyes in congenital syphilis.

W. Hector and G. H. Fairley, *Textbook of Medicine for Nurses*, 2nd edn, Heinemann, 1973. Chapter 14 (pp. 353, 389) describes some of the disorders of the optic nerves and the conditions which cause them.

A. King and C. Nicol, *Venereal Diseases*, 2nd edn, Baillière, Tindall & Cassell, 1969. Chapter 6 (pp. 84–6) gives a clear account of interstitial keratitis in congenital syphilis.

D. McAlpine, C. E. Lumsden and E. D. Acheson, *Multiple Sclerosis: A Reappraisal*, 2nd edn, Churchill Livingstone, 1972. Chapter 5 (pp. 148–63) provides a detailed account of the way multiple sclerosis affects the eye. Good for more advanced students, though not for beginners.

J. Malins, *Clinical Diabetes Mellitus*, Eyre & Spottiswoode, 1968. Chapter 8 (pp. 186–207) gives a clear, detailed account of the pathology, causes, treatment and management of defects in the eye in diabetes.

M. Mason and H. L. F. Currey (eds.), *An Introduction to Clinical Rheumatology*, Pitman Medical, 1970. Includes brief accounts of the connection between the disease and the eye, e.g. the eye in rheumatoid arthritis (p. 27), ocular involvement in ankylosing spondylitis (p. 55) and an account of Sjögren's syndrome (chapter 10).

W. G. Oakley, D. A. Pyke and K. W. Taylor, *Diabetes and its Management*, Blackwell, 1973. Chapter 10 (pp. 109–17) describes the eye in diabetes: the disorders which may arise in each part of the eye – how they are caused, their prevention and treatment with clear illustrations of the conditions.

P. D. Trevor-Roper, *Lecture Notes on Ophthalmology*, 4th edn, Blackwell, 1971. Several useful sections: p. 46 lists diseases including acute iritis, p. 52 outlines acute keratitis and its endogenous causes, p. 55 describes the relationship between interstitial keratitis and congenital syphilis, p. 62 gives causes of secondary cataract, p. 70 gives some causes of optic neuritis and compression and p. 75 describes renal and diabetic retinopathy.

Chapter 4
Books

W. P. Gowland and J. Cairney, *Anatomy and Physiology for Nurses*, 7th edn, Peryer, Christchurch, New Zealand, 1965. Chapter 12 (pp. 238–42) describes the senses of smell and taste, the nose, nasal sinuses and tongue.

S. Marshall and Z. Oxlade, *Ear, Nose and Throat Nursing*, 5th edn, Baillière Tindall, 1972. Section 2 describes the nose and accessory sinuses.

J. S. Ross and K. Wilson, *Foundations of Anatomy and Physiology*, 3rd edn, Churchill Livingstone, 1968. Chapter 9 (pp. 197–9) describes the structure of of the nose and nasal cavities, while chapter 16 (pp. 426–43) deals with the nose and the physiology of smell.

Articles

M. E. Gibb, 'Epistaxis', *Nursing Times*, vol. 67, 6 April 1971, pp. 403–5. The causes, clinical features and immediate treatment. How to pack the nose – other methods of treatment, e.g. cauterization and ligature of vessels.

N. Shah, 'ENT emergencies: 1 Epistaxis', *Nursing Mirror*, vol. 136, 10 March 1972, pp. 28–30. Classification of causes of nose bleeding and methods of treatment.

N. Shah, 'ENT emergencies: 2 Foreign bodies in ENT', *Nursing Mirror*, vol. 134, 17 March 1972, pp. 39–41. Includes treatment of foreign bodies in the nose and air passages.

Chapter 5
Books

S. Marshall and Z. Oxlade, *Ear, Nose and Throat Nursing*, 5th edn, Baillière Tindall, 1972. Section 2 deals with the accessory sinuses.

J. S. Ross and K. Wilson, *Foundations of Anatomy and Physiology*, 3rd edn, Churchill Livingstone, 1968. Chapter 9 (pp. 197–9) describes the structure of the nose and nasal cavities.

Articles

A. G. Gibbs, 'Antral puncture', *Nursing Times*, vol. 67, 15 July 1971, pp. 851–2. The requirements, methods and complications of the procedure – with common pitfalls for the nurse.

O. H. Shaheen, 'Disorders of the sinuses', *Nursing Times*, vol. 69, 24 May 1973, pp. 673–4. Types of sinusitis, the symptoms and treatment.

Chapter 6
Books

W. P. Gowland and J. Cairney, *Anatomy and Physiology for Nurses*, 7th edn, Peryer, Christchurch, New Zealand, 1965. Chapter 12 (pp. 238–42) includes the sense of taste and the tongue.

J. S. Ross and K. Wilson, *Foundations of Anatomy and Physiology*, 3rd edn, Churchill Livingstone, 1968. Chapter 16 (pp. 426–43) includes the tongue and the physiology of taste.

Articles

W. Henderson, 'Complications of infections of the mouth and pharynx in children', *Nursing Times*, vol. 68, 11 May 1972, pp. 569–70. Some of the complications which may occur in children who do not complain of their sore throats.

C. Smith, 'Infections of the mouth and pharynx', *Nursing Times*, vol. 68, 11 May 1972, pp. 566–8. Examination of the mouth and pharynx. Some acute infections, their diagnosis and treatment.

B. G. Wood and G. A. Kevill, 'Nursing care of babies with cleft lip and palate: 1 The Pierre Robin Syndrome', *Nursing Times*, vol. 66, 29 Oct. 1970, pp. 1385–9. How this arises – manifestations at birth. Management handling and feeding of the baby prior to surgical treatment at fourteen months.

B. G. Wood and G. A. Kevill, 'Nursing care of babies with cleft lip and palate: 2 Presurgical correction of the deformed maxillary arch', *Nursing Times*, vol. 66, 5 Nov. 1970, pp. 1420–25. Origin of the deformity – immediate correction at birth by means of acrylic feeding plate, then appliance in the mouth to help correction of maxillary arch. Handling of baby and mother. Lip and palate closure at a later date.

B. G. Wood, 'Nursing care of babies with cleft lip and palate: 3 Trisomy of the 13–15 chromosome group (Patau's Syndrome – trisomy D I)', *Nursing Times*, vol. 66, 12 Nov. 1970, pp. 1459–61. Appearance of this abnormality at birth. Case study of a baby who died after 34 days.

B. G. Wood and G. A. Kevill, 'Nursing care of babies with cleft lip and palate: 4 The immediate pre- and post-operative nursing care', *Nursing Times*, vol. 66, 19 Nov. 1970, pp. 1490–93. Detailed account of operations performed with pre- and post-operative care needed.

Chapter 7
Books

S. Marshall and Z. Oxlade, *Ear, Nose and Throat Nursing*, Baillière Tindall, 1972. Section 3 deals with the pharynx: anatomy of the pharynx, diseases of the throat, tonsillectomy and adenoidectomy. Section 4 deals with the larynx, trachea and oesophagus: anatomy of the larynx, voice production, and swallowing, diseases of the larynx, operations on the larynx and pharynx, foreign bodies and endoscopy.

Articles

C. Brown, 'Nursing care study: total laryngectomy', *Nursing Times*, vol. 67, 16 Sept. 1971, pp. 1144–7. An account of the pre- and post-operative care of an elderly man having laryngectomy. How difficulties of eating, breathing and communication were overcome.

W. Henderson, 'Complications of the mouth and pharynx in children', *Nursing Times*, vol. 68, 11 May 1972, pp. 569–70. Some of the complications which may occur in children who do not complain of sore throats.

G. Russell, 'Acute epiglottitis in children', *Nursing Times*, vol. 69, 8 March 1973, pp. 306–8. An account of the serious nature of this disorder in producing laryngeal obstruction. Comparison with other causes of obstruction – with treatment.

N. Shah, 'ENT emergencies: 2 Foreign bodies in ENT', *Nursing Mirror*, vol. 134, 17 March 1972, pp. 39–41. Includes treatment of foreign bodies in the pharynx and oesophagus.

N. Shah, 'ENT emergencies: 4 Respiratory obstruction and tracheostomy', *Nursing Mirror*, vol. 134, 31 March 1972, pp. 35–8. List of causes of respiratory obstruction. Effects and treatment of tracheostomy, the operation and tubes, and post-operative care.

C. Smith, 'Infections of the mouth and pharynx', *Nursing Times*, vol. 68, 11 May 1972, pp. 566–8. Examination of the mouth and pharynx. Some acute infections, their diagnosis and treatment.

Chapters 8 and 9
Books

J. C. Ballantyne, *Deafness*, 2nd edn, Churchill Livingstone, 1970. An account of deafness as it affects people of all ages and in its medical, educational, psychological and social aspects.

P. H. Beales, *Noise, Hearing and Deafness*, Michael Joseph, 1965. Normal hearing, causes of deafness and its medical and surgical treatment. Education and welfare of the deaf.

W. P. Gowland and J. Cairney, *Anatomy and Physiology for Nurses*, 7th edn, Peryer, Christchurch, New Zealand. Chapter 12 (pp. 230–37) describes the structure and function of the ear, and hearing.

G. L. McCulloch, *Man Alive: A Survey of Human Physiology*, Aldus, 1967. Chapter 9 (pp. 106–9) gives an illustrated account of the structure and function of the ear.

S. Marshall and Z. Oxlade, *Ear, Nose and Throat Nursing*, 5th edn, Baillière Tindall, 1972. Section 5 deals with the ear: anatomy and physiology, deafness, diseases of the external, middle and inner ear, and operations on the ear.

National Institute for the Deaf, *The Deaf in Britain: A General Outline*, The Institute, 1961. Classification of deafness. Treatment and welfare at all ages pre-school, schooling, training for work and placement. Methods of communication.

S. Ross and K. Wilson, *Foundations of Anatomy and Physiology*, 3rd edn, Churchill Livingstone, 1968. Chapter 16 includes the structure and function of the ear.

T. H. Sutcliffe, *Deafness – Let's Face It*, Church of England Council for the Deaf, 1970. The problem of deafness, its effects on personality and everyday activity. Hearing aids, education of deaf children, general welfare, etc.

Articles

E. M. Andrews, 'Understanding the world of deaf children', *Nursing Mirror*, vol. 126, 24 May 1968, pp. 38–9. The work of the audiometric health visitor.

R. W. Bailie, 'Deafness – a problem of communication', *Nursing Times*, vol. 68, 27 July 1972, pp. 923–6. Mechanisms of hearing. Incidence and grading of deafness – its investigation and management.

B. H. Colman, 'Chronic mucous otitis', *Nursing Times*, vol. 69, 15 March 1973, pp. 336–8. An account of the causes, pathology, diagnosis and treatment of the condition.

M. R. Dix, 'Hearing tests in modern clinical practice', *Nursing Mirror*, vol. 128, 28 Feb. 1969, pp. 30–35. New test procedures for the accurate measurement of hearing pure-tone audiograms, speech audiograms, peep-show audiometry, etc.

R. Edwards, 'Deafness in children: 4 What it means to be deaf – and the educational facilities we are providing', *Nursing Times*, vol. 64, 20 Dec. 1968, pp. 1718–20. Effects of deafness. Details of the range of facilities available. Educational provision in Northern Ireland.

R. Edwards, 'Deafness in children: 5 Helping them to help their children', *Nursing Times*, vol. 64, 27 Dec. 1968, pp. 1759–61. Guidance for parents of deaf children. The ways in which they can supplement the statutory help given.

R. Edwards, 'Deafness in children: 6 Deaf not dumb – teaching deaf children to speak', *Nursing Times*, vol. 65, 2 Jan. 1969, pp. 12–14. Methods used by the teachers of deaf children.

L. Fisch, 'Causes of congenital deafness', *Public Health*, vol. 83, Jan. 1969, pp. 68–74. A study of a number of cases of deafness showing the different causes.

A. G. Gibbs, 'Syringing the ear', *Nursing Times*, vol. 66, 1 Oct. 1970, pp. 1264–6. Indication and contra-indication. How to soften wax, lotions to use, types of syringe and technique. Some complications.

A. G. Gibbs, 'Tympanoplasty', *Nursing Times*, vol. 64, 25 Oct. 1968, pp. 1434–7. The ear and mechanism of hearing. Principles of tympanoplasty – details of operations performed with outline of after-treatment.

R. M. Harvey, 'Deafness in children: 1 The causes', *Nursing Times*, vol. 64, 29 Nov. 1968, pp. 1623–5. Effect of deafness on a child, causes of deafness from birth and early childhood.

R. M. Harvey, 'Deafness in children: 2 How deaf?', *Nursing Times*, vol. 64, 6 Dec. 1968, pp. 1659–61. Methods of testing deafness in children.

R. M. Harvey, 'Deafness in children: 3 Treatment', *Nursing Times*, vol. 64, 13 Dec. 1968, pp. 1694–5. Methods of treatment: hearing aids, operative measures, elimination of infection.

J. D. Kershaw, 'The audiology revolution', *Public Health*, vol. 87, May 1973, pp. 99–105. The aetiology of hearing disability, its assessment and treatment. The approach to deafness in the education of deaf children.

J. M. McCauley, 'Nursing care in microsurgery of the ear', *Nursing Times*, vol. 65, 20 March 1969, pp. 361–2. A brief account of the special nursing required.

W. McKenzie, 'Stapes surgery', *Nursing Mirror*, vol. 113, 10 Feb. 1967, pp. 1–3. Past operations to restore hearing. A detailed account of modern stapendectomy and its value.

S. Mawson, 'Problem of the born-deaf child', *Nursing Mirror*, vol. 126, 26 April 1968, pp. 30–31. Importance of early recognition; early medical treatment and auditory training.

R. S. Olomon, 'They don't always speak', *Nursing Times*, vol. 65, 10 July 1959, pp. 896–7. The plight of the totally deaf – communication based on sign language.

H. M. Parsons, 'Surgery for diseases of the mastoid process', *Nursing Times*, vol. 66, 23 July 1970, pp. 942–5. Different types of operation are discussed with some of the reasons for their choice.

G. D. L. Smyth, 'Microsurgical treatment for deafness', *Nursing Times*, vol. 65, 20 March 1969, pp. 359–61. A review of some of the surgical advances in the treatment of deafness, including stapendectomy and tympanoplasty.

E. C. N. Strong, 'Deafness in the elderly' (based on a talk given at RCN course in Birmingham in 1969), *Nursing Mirror*, vol. 129, 11 July 1969, pp. 19–21 and 18 July 1969, pp. 50–51. Why the elderly become deaf. Their main hearing problems – what can be done to help them. Hearing aids.

Acknowledgements

We wish to thank the following for permission to use material that has been the basis for some of the illustrations.

For Figures 5, 85 and 94: Orbis Publishing Company, *Mind and Body*. For Figures 12, 24, 30, 34 and 36; Blackwell Scientific Publications Ltd, *Ophthalmology* by P. D. Trevor-Roper. For Figures 14, 25 and 29: Faber & Faber Ltd, *Ophthalmic Nursing* by P. Garland. For Figure 26: Queen Victoria Hospital, East Grinstead. For Figure 33: Churchill Livingstone, *Illustrated Physiology* by A. B. McNaught and R. R. Callender. For Figure 40: J. & A. Churchill, *Anatomy* by T. Gray. For Figures 60, 61, 78, 81, 84, 86b and 93: Baillière Tindall: *Ear, Nose and Throat Nursing* by S. Marshall and Z. Oxlade. For Figure 62: Baillière Tindall, *Diseases of the Nose and Throat* by Sir S. Clair Thompson and V. E. Negus. For Figure 69: Churchill Livingstone, *Textbook of Operative Surgery* by E. L. Farquharson. For Figures 80 and 92: Butterworth & Co. Ltd, *Diseases of the Ear, Nose and Throat* by John Ballantyne and John Groves.

Figures 6, 9, 11, 13, 22b, 27, 28, 79, 82, 91 and 93: photographs by Peter G. Tucker. Figures 15, 17 and 18: photographs courtesy Queen Victoria Hospital, East Grinstead. Figures 16, 19, 20, 21, 22a, 23, 25, 31, 32 and 38: photographs courtesy Hillingdon Hospital.

Index